ISCHEMIC PRECONDITIONING: THE CONCEPT OF ENDOGENOUS CARDIOPROTECTION

DEVELOPMENTS IN CARDIOVASCULAR MEDICINE

S. Sideman, R. Beyar and A. G. Kleber (eds.): Cardiac Electrophysiology, Circulation, and Transport. Proceedings of the 7th Henry Goldberg Workshop (Berne, Switzerland, 1990). 1991. ISBN 0-7923-1145-0.
D. M. Bers: Excitation-Contraction Coupling and Cardiac Contractile Force. 1991. ISBN 0-7923-1186-8.
A.-M. Salmasi and A. N. Nicolaides (eds.): Occult Atherosclerotic Disease. Diagnosis, Assessment and Management. 1991. ISBN 0-7923-1188-4.
J. A. E. Spaan: Coronary Blood Flow. Mechanics, Distribution, and Control. 1991. ISBN 0-7923-1210-4.
R. W. Stout (ed.): Diabetes and Atherosclerosis. 1991. ISBN 0-7923-1310-0.
A. G. Herman (ed.): Antithrombotics. Pathophysiological Rationale for Pharmacological Interventions. 1991. ISBN 0-7923-1413-1.
N. H. J. Pijls: Maximal Myocardial Perfusion as a Measure of the Functional Significance of Coronary Arteriogram. From a Pathoanatomic to a Pathophysiologic Interpretation of the Coronary Arteriogram. 1991. ISBN 0-7923-1430-1.
J. H. C. Reiber and E. E. v. d. Wall (eds.): Cardiovascular Nuclear Medicine and MRI. Quantitation and Clinical Applications. 1992. ISBN 0-7923-1467-0.
E. Andries, P. Brugada and R. Stroobrandt (eds.): How to Face "the Faces" of Cardiac Pacing. 1992. ISBN 0-7923-1528-6.
M. Nagano, S. Mochizuki and N. S. Dhalla (eds.): Cardiovascular Disease in Diabetes. 1992. ISBN 0-7923-1554-5.
P. W. Serruys, B. H. Strauss and S. B. King III (eds.): Restenosis after Intervention with New Mechanical Devices. 1992. ISBN 0-7923-1555-3.
P. J. Winter (ed.): Quality of Life after Open Heart Surgery. 1992. ISBN 0-7923-1580-4.
E. E. van der Wall, H. Sochot, A. Righetti and M. G. Niemeyer (eds.): What is new in Cardiac Imaging? SPECT, PET and MRI. 1992. ISBN 0-7923-1615-0.
P. Hanrath, R. Uebis and W. Krebs (eds.): Cardiovascular Imaging by Ultrasound. 1992. ISBN 0-7923-1755-6.
F. H. Messerli (ed.): Cardiovascular Disease in the Elderly, 3rd ed. 1992. ISBN 0-7923-1859-5.
J. Hess and G. R. Sutherland (eds.): Congenital Heart Disease in Adolescents and Adults. 1992. ISBN 0-7923-1862-5.
J. H. C. Reiber and P. W. Serruys (eds.): Advances in Quantitative Coronary Arteriography. 1992. ISBN 0-7923-1863-3.
A.-M. Salmasi and A. S. Iskandrian (eds.): Cardiac Output and Regional Flow in Health and Disease. 1993. ISBN 0-7923-1911-7.
J. H. Kingma, N. M. van Hemel and K. I. Lie (eds.): Atrial Fibrillation, a Treatable Disease? 1992. ISBN 0-7923-2008-5.
B. Ostadal, N. S. Dhalla (eds.): Heart Function in Health and Disease. 1993. ISBN 0-7923-2052-2.
D. Noble and Y. E. Earm (eds.): Ionic Channels and Effect of Taurine on the Heart. Proceedings of an International Symposium (Seoul, Korea, 1992). 1993. ISBN 0-7923-2199-5.
H. M. Piper (ed.): Ischemia-reperfusion in Cardiac Surgery. 1993. ISBN 0-7923-2241-X.

ISCHEMIC PRECONDITIONING: THE CONCEPT OF ENDOGENOUS CARDIOPROTECTION

Edited by
KARIN PRZYKLENK
ROBERT A. KLONER
The Heart Institute
The Hospital of the Good Samaritan
Los Angeles, CA

DEREK M. YELLON
Department of Academic Cardiology
University College Hospital
London, United Kingdom

SPRINGER SCIENCE+BUSINESS MEDIA, LLC

Originally published by Kluwer Academic Publishers in 1994

Printed on acid-free paper.

Library of Congress Cataloging-in-Publication Data

Ischemic preconditioning: the concept of endogenous
cardioprotection / edited by Karin Przyklenk, Robert A. Kloner and Derek M. Yellon.
p. cm. — (Developments in cardiovascular medicine; DICM 148)
Includes index.
ISBN 978-0-7923-2410-2 ISBN 978-1-4615-2602-5 (eBook)
DOI 10.1007/978-1-4615-2602-5
1. Myocardial infarction—Prevention. 2. Coronary heart disease. 3. Heart—Adaptation. I. Przyklenk, Karin, 1956– . II. Kloner, Robert A. III. Yellon, Derek M. IV. Series. V. Series: Developments in cardiovascular medicine; v. 148.
[DNLM: 1. Myocardial Ischemia. 2. Myocardial Diseases—prevention & control. 3. Adaptation, Physiological. W1 DE997VME v. 148]
RC685.I6I83 1993
616.1'23—dc20
DNLM/DLC
for Library of Congress 93-21904
CIP

CONTENTS

LIST OF CONTRIBUTORS

John A. Auchampach, PhD
Postdoctoral Fellow
Cardiovascular Diseases Research and Adhesion Biology
The Upjohn Company
301 Henrietta Street
Kalamazoo, MI 49001

Barbara Bauer, MD
Department of Cardiology
Medizinische Universitätsklinik Würzburg
Josef Schneider Strasse 2
Bau 4
Luitpoldkrankenhaus
8700 Würzburg
Germany

James M. Downey, PhD
Professor of Physiology
Department of Medical Physiology
University of South Alabama
MSB 3024
Mobile, AL 36688

Garrett J. Gross, PhD
Professor of Pharmacology and Toxicology
Department of Pharmacology and Toxicology
Medical College of Wisconsin
8701 Watertown Plank Road
Milwaukee, WI 53226

Richard J. Heads
Research Fellow
The Hatter Institute for Cardiovascular Studies
Department of Academic Cardiology
University College Hospital
Gower Street
London WC1E 6AU
United Kingdom

Prof. David J. Hearse, PhD DSc
Director of Research
Cardiovascular Research
The Rayne Institute
St. Thomas' Hospital
London SE1 7EH
United Kingdom

Robert B. Jennings, MD
James B. Duke Professor of Pathology
Department of Pathology
Box 3712
Duke University Medical Center
Durham, NC 27710

Robert A. Kloner, MD, PhD
Director of Research
Heart Institute, Hospital of the Good Samaritan
Professor of Medicine, Section of Cardiology
University of Southern California
616 South Witmer Street
Los Angeles, CA 90017

Clive S. Lawson, MRCP
Registrar in Cardiology
The London Chest Hospital
Bonner Road
London E2 9JX
United Kingdom

Yongge Liu
Department of Medical Physiology
University of South Alabama
MSB 3024
Mobile, AL 36688

Michael S. Marber, MRCP
Honorary Senior Registrar in Cardiology
British Heart Foundation Intermediate Fellow
The Hatter Institute for Cardiovascular Studies
Department of Academic Cardiology
University College Hospital
Gower Street
London WC1E 6AU
United Kingdom

Charles E. Murry, MD, PhD
Acting Instructor in Pathology
Department of Pathology
RC-72
University of Washington Medical Center
Seattle, WA 98135

Michel Ovize, MD
Adjunct Assistant Professor
Department of Cardiology
Hopital Cardiologique Louis Pradel
Service du Pr. J. Delaye
59, Boulevard Pinel
69003 Lyon
France

Karin Przyklenk, PhD
Assistant Director of Research and Director of Cardiac Function
Heart Institute, Hospital of the Good Samaritan
Associate Professor of Research Medicine, Section of Cardiology
University of Southern California
616 South Witmer Street
Los Angeles, CA 90017

Keith A. Reimer, MD, PhD
Professor of Pathology
Head, Cardiovascular Pathology
Department of Pathology
Box 3712
Duke University Medical Center
Durham, NC 27710

Richard S. Vander Heide, MD
Cardiac Pathology Fellow
Department of Pathology
Box 3712
Duke University Medical Center
Durham, NC 27710

Peter Whittaker, PhD
Director of Microscopy
Heart Institute/Hospital of the Good Samaritan
Assistant Professor of Research Medicine
University of Southern California
616 South Witmer Street
Los Angeles, CA 90017

Zhenhai Yao, MD
Visiting Scientist
Department of Pharmacology and Toxicology
Medical College of Wisconsin
8701 Watertown Plank Road
Milwaukee, WI 53226

Derek M. Yellon, PhD
Professor of Cellular Cardiology
Head of Division of Cardiology
Director, The Hatter Institute for Cardiovascular Studies
Department of Academic Cardiology
University College Hospital
Gower Street
London WC1E 6AU
United Kingdom

Kirsti Ytrehus, MD, PhD
Assistant Professor of Physiology
Department of Physiology
University of Tromso
Tromso, Norway
[Currently on sabbatical in
Department of Medical Physiology
University of South Alabama
MSB 3024
Mobile, AL 36688

PREFACE

In 1985, Murry and colleagues provided the first preliminary evidence that repeated brief episodes of coronary artery occlusion protected the canine myocardium and limited infarct size caused by subsequent sustained ischemia. This paradoxical concept of endogenous, ischemia-induced cardioprotection, termed *ischemic "preconditioning"*, has become a focus of attention for investigators involved in all aspects of myocardial ischemia and reperfusion. In fact, a survey of abstracts presented on this topic at the Scientific Sessions of the American Heart Association (Figure 1) reveals the burgeoning interest of the worldwide scientific community in this cardioprotective phenomenon.

Subsequent to this seminal report, infarct size reduction with ischemic preconditioning has been observed to occur in a host of in vivo experimental models, including the dog, rabbit, rat, and pig. Furthermore, recent clinical evidence suggests that brief episodes of coronary occlusion may also increase the tolerance to subsequent ischemia in patients during angioplasty procedures. While these data leave no doubt that preconditioning can limit infarct size, three crucial questions concerning this phenomenon remain unresolved. The first and obvious unanswered question is *what are the cause(s) or mechanism(s) responsible for this protective effect?* Secondly, *do the benefits of ischemic preconditioning extend beyond the concept of myocyte viability and attenuate other deleterious sequelae associated with sustained ischemia/reperfusion?* Finally, *does the phenomenon of ischemic preconditioning occur clinically* and, perhaps most importantly, *can preconditioning be used as a therapeutic tool in patients with*

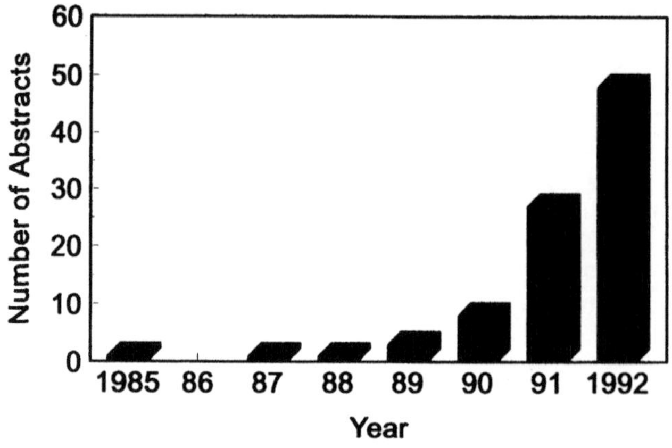

Figure 1. Abstracts on preconditioning presented at the AHA scientific sessions.

ischemic syndromes (including acute myocardial infarction), and in patients undergoing coronary bypass surgery?

Our objective in compiling this monograph is to consolidate, in one volume, both the current knowledge and most recent advances on the subject of ischemic preconditioning. To this end, we have solicited investigators at the forefront of ongoing research to provide their scholarly and candid comments concerning each of these issues. Specifically, we include a comprehensive review of infarct size reduction with ischemic preconditioning and the most recent data on the effects of preconditioning on ischemia- and reperfusion-induced arrhythmias, myocardial metabolism, contractile function, and the coronary vasculature. The role of altered energy metabolism, stress-induced proteins, ATP-sensitive potassium channels, and adenosine — the major hypotheses that have been proposed to explain the cardioprotective effects of ischemic preconditioning — are critically reviewed by investigators who have been instrumental in developing these concepts. In addition, we raise the intriguing possibility that ischemic preconditioning may be more than simply a laboratory curiosity. Using a multidisciplinary approach, we aim to inform the reader of the "facts" of ischemic preconditioning, and to challenge the reader to contribute their own expertise to address the unanswered questions concerning this endogenous, cardioprotective phenomenon.

ACKNOWLEDGMENTS

First and foremost, we express our appreciation to the colleagues and friends who have provided expert contributions to this text.

Many of the concepts discussed in the following chapters were convened at a unique round-table meeting at Hanbury Manor, United Kingdom, in October 1992, held under the auspices of the Council on Cardiac Metabolism of the International Society and Federation of Cardiology. We are grateful to Gensia Europe for providing an educational grant both to sponsor the round-table meeting and to support the publication of this book.

We thank the members of the board of directors and administration of both the Heart Institute, Hospital of the Good Samaritan, and Hatter Institute for Cardiovascular Studies for providing the fertile academic environments that enable us to pursue our research and educational endeavors. Finally, we appreciate the patience and unfailing support of our families throughout the preparation of this book.

Karin Przyklenk
Robert A. Kloner
Derek M. Yellon

I. ISCHEMIC PRECONDITIONING: BENEFITS AND LIMITATIONS IN EXPERIMENTAL MODELS OF ISCHEMIA/REPERFUSION

1. WHAT IS ISCHEMIC PRECONDITIONING?

CHARLES E. MURRY, ROBERT B. JENNINGS, and KEITH A. REIMER

INTRODUCTION

In the last 10 years our understanding of the heart's response to ischemic injury has changed dramatically. Until the mid-1980s, prevailing opinion held that reversibly injured myocardium was more vulnerable to the effects of a subsequent period of ischemia [1,2]. Cardiac biologists considered tissue injured by, for example, a 15-minute period of ischemia, to remain near the brink of cell death for many hours after it was salvaged by reperfusion. This notion turned out to be wrong; in fact, the exact opposite is true. Paradoxically, myocardium that has been reversibly injured by ischemia is *more tolerant* of a subsequent episode of ischemia. This phenomenon has been termed *ischemic preconditioning* [3]. In this chapter we shall describe the studies that led to our original report of the preconditioning phenomenon and review the effects of preconditioning on myocardial infarct size. We shall then review the effects of repeated, brief ischemic insults in other organs and compare their responses with that of the heart.

DEFINITIONS, EXPERIMENTAL END POINTS, AND MODEL SYSTEMS

We originally defined preconditioning as a *rapid, adaptive response to a brief ischemic insult, which slowed the rate of cell death during a subsequent, prolonged period of ischemia* [3]. Several points are important in this definition: (1) It is induced by ischemia, (2) the response is rapid (minutes), and (3) it is manifest as a limitation of cell death. Subsequent studies have extended the term *preconditioning* to include adaptation to stimuli other than ischemia, such as heat shock [4,5], various drug treatments [e.g., 6], and mechanical stretch [7]. Furthermore, the term also has been applied to various end points that were not contemplated in the original definition. These include dysrhythmias [8,9], contractile function [10], autonomic nerve conduction [11], and vasomotor function [12] in both in vivo and in isolated heart preparations. Although these phenomena appear similar on initial examination, we stress that they may not be manifestations of ischemic preconditioning as originally defined.

This distinction is more than academic. For example, although limitation of infarct size by a drug is a prerequisite for it to induce the same pathway as preconditioning, it is not sufficient evidence to conclude that they operate by the same mechanism. The same caveat applies to other interventions, such as heat shock or mechanical stretch: A similar end point does not indicate a similar means. Conversely, although a preconditioning protocol may attenuate dysrhythmias during a subsequent prolonged period of ischemia, this result may be mediated by an entirely different mechanism than the limitation of infarct size. In studies of isolated, buffer perfused hearts the most commonly used end point is postischemic contractile dysfunction. In most of these studies, however, postischemic dysfunction is the summation of both lethal injury and dysfunction of viable cells (stunning). When both are present it is very difficult to determine which component has been affected by preconditioning. Thus, simply lumping these different models and end points into one generic category could result in long-term confusion.

To avoid such confusion, until we know more about how these various adaptive changes take place, we propose that investigators studying *preconditioning*, *endogenous cardioprotection*, or whatever term one chooses to apply, should clearly distinguish (1) the means of inducing the adaptation, (2) the experimental end point, and (3) the species and model used for study.

BACKGROUND STUDIES LEADING TO PRECONDITIONING

Effects of repeated brief episodes of ischemia

A longstanding goal in myocardial ischemia research has been to determine the biochemical events that lead to irreversible cell injury. The metabolic consequences of ischemia can be classified under two general headings: depletion of high energy phosphates and the accumulation of ischemic catabolites. In the late 1970s and early 1980s studies were done that implicated both severe depletion of adenosine triphosphate (ATP) [13] and accumulation of glycolytic intermediates [14] in the pathogenesis of lethal ischemic cell injury. Although it seems clear that the two components have additive deleterious effects, it is somewhat surprising that we still do not know in precise terms the relative contributions of each to cell death.

The studies that led to preconditioning were based on several reports from the early 1980s, which demonstrated that ATP resynthesis after a single episode of ischemia was very slow, taking as much as 4 days to recover after a 15-minute coronary occlusion [15–17]. The delayed metabolic recovery raised the possibility that repeated, brief episodes of ischemia (such as occur with angina pectoris) might cause cumulative ATP depletion and eventually result in myocardial necrosis. This presented, we thought, an excellent opportunity to dissociate the effects of ATP depletion from catabolite accumulation. We reasoned that while repeated ischemic episodes would induce a cumulative, "stair-step" depletion of ATP, the intermittent reperfusion would wash out ischemic catabolites.

Based on these premises, two separate but related experiments were begun in parallel. In one experiment we studied the effects of repeated 10-minute coronary occlusions to test whether repeated ischemic events, by themselves insufficient to cause lethal injury, would cause a cumulative depletion of ATP and cell death. In the other experiment we studied the effects of antecedent brief episodes of ischemia on cell death after a sustained occlusion, which by itself would normally cause substantial myocardial necrosis. In the repeated 10-minute occlusion study, we were very surprised to learn that four 10-minute coronary occlusions caused no more ATP depletion than a single occlusion; in other words, there was no cumulative metabolic effect [18]. This finding indicated a slowing of ATP depletion in subsequent ischemic episodes, which we determined was due to a marked slowing of the rate of ATP utilization. As one would then predict, four 10-minute occlusions caused virtually no myocardial necrosis, despite the fact that 40 minutes of sustained ischemia typically produces a confluent subendocardial infarction. Similar metabolic data were reported by several other groups as well [19–22]. These studies demonstrated that repeated, brief ischemic insults did not have the cumulative impact of a sustained ischemic episode. We concluded that intermittent reperfusion prevented cumulative injury by washing out ischemic catabolites, recharging high energy phosphate pools, and restoring the capacity for anaerobic glycolysis during subsequent occlusions.

Demonstrating that preconditioning limits infarct size

After completing the repeated 10-minute occlusion studies we still did not know how reversibly injured myocardium would respond to a prolonged period of ischemia, one that normally would result in a substantial amount of cell death. As mentioned above, we were attempting to test this hypothesis concurrently with the 10-minute occlusion study but were delayed by major technical problems. Our initial efforts used two 10-minute occlusions of the proximal circumflex artery, followed by a sustained 40-minute test occlusion. This protocol caused intractable ventricular fibrillation in about 75% of the experiments, generally during the second period of ischemia or reperfusion. Making matters worse, the surviving animals had relatively high collateral

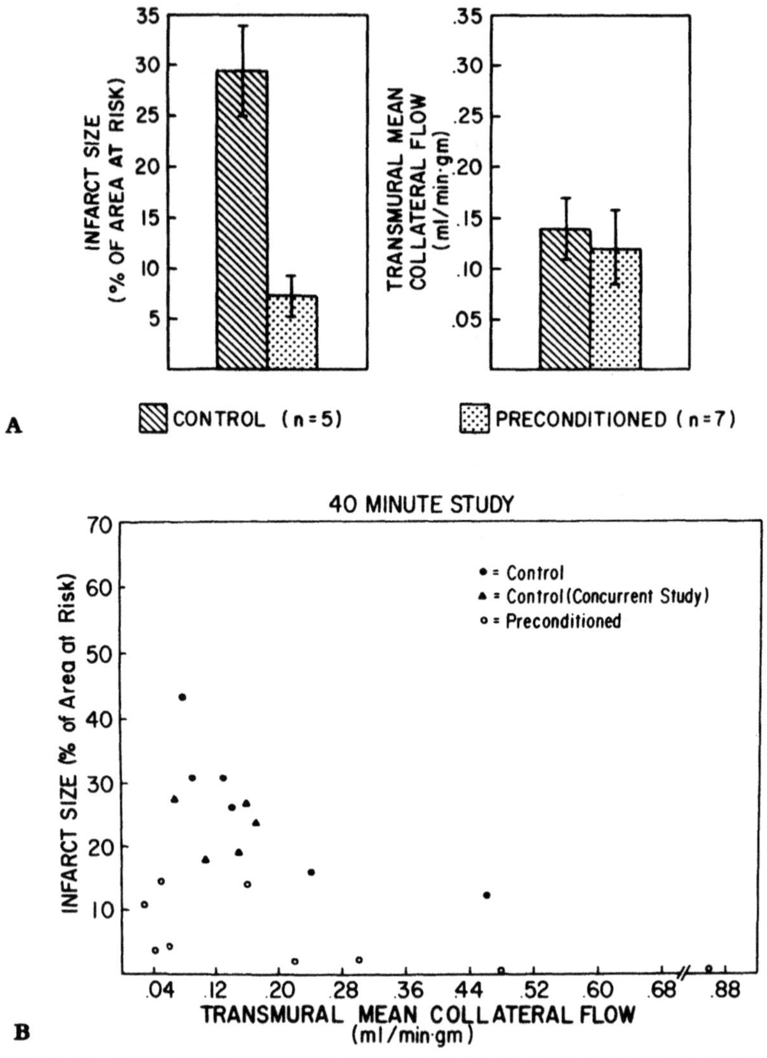

Figure 1. **A:** Bar graph showing effects of preconditioning on myocardial infarct size in dogs. Dogs were preconditioned with four 5-minute occlusion of the proximal circumflex artery, each separated by 5 minutes of reperfusion. They were then subjected to a sustained 40-minute ischemic episode. Control animals received a single 40-minute circumflex occlusion. Infarcts were sized histologically after 4 days reperfusion and related to anatomic area at risk and collateral blood flow (measured with radioactive microspheres midway through the sustained occlusion). In control animals infarct size averaged 29% of the area at risk. In preconditioned animals, infarct size was markedly smaller, averaging 7% of the area at risk. Collateral blood flow to the ischemic region was not significantly different between groups. Reproduced from Murry et al. [3], by permission. **B:** Regression of infarct size vs. collateral blood flow. In control animals there was an inverse relation between infarct size and collateral blood flow, i.e., low flow was associated with large infarcts and vice versa. In preconditioned animals infarcts were much smaller than controls at any level of collateral blood flow. Reproduced from Murry et al. [3], by permission.

blood flows and would not have been expected to develop significant infarcts in any case. We then attempted to use a single 10-minute circumflex occlusion, followed by a 40-minute sustained occlusion, and again had an unacceptably high incidence of ventricular fibrillation. Attempts to reduce the incidence of fibrillation with the antiarrhythmic drug bretylium tosylate were similarly unsuccessful. These failures led us to the conclusion that a 10-minute circumflex occlusion increased the heart's susceptibility to ventricular fibrillation.

Based on the metabolic findings of the repeated 10-minute occlusion study (which were by this time completed), we knew that brief episodes of ischemia changed the rate of ATP consumption during ischemia. We thought that this could have a significant impact on cell death during a sustained episode of ischemia and therefore felt compelled to find a protocol that permitted us to test this hypothesis. Our subsequent efforts were more successful [3]. We subjected the myocardium to four 5-minute coronary occlusions, each separated by 5 minutes of reperfusion. This protocol was chosen empirically to provide the cumulative ischemic time of the original protocol of two 10-minute occlusion; 5-minute reperfusion periods were chosen because that is close to the minimum time required to achieve complete washout of ischemic catabolites and restoration of the adenylate charge [23]. This protocol not only eliminated the problem of fibrillation, but also markedly limited the size of infarcts resulting from a sustained 40-minute occlusion. Control animals had infarcts of 29% of the area at risk, while preconditioned animals had infarcts averaging only 7% of the area at risk (Figure 1). This marked limitation of infarct size was not due to increased collateral perfusion; collateral blood flow, measured with radioactive microspheres midway through the 40-minute occlusion, was not significantly different between the control and preconditioned groups.

PRECONDITIONING CAN BE ACHIEVED WITH MULTIPLE PROTOCOLS AND IN MULTIPLE SPECIES

Many other laboratories have subsequently verified the protective effects of preconditioning. Although we originally used four 5-minute coronary occlusions in dogs, there is general agreement that preconditioning can be induced with a variety of protocols and in multiple species. Single occlusions of 2.5, 5, or 15 minutes have been shown to be protective in dogs [24–26]. In our experience (KA Reimer, unpublished observations), the shortest single occlusion to induce preconditioning in dogs is 90 seconds. One 5-minute or two 2-minute occlusions are sufficient to precondition rabbit myocardium [27,28]. Swine myocardium has been preconditioned with two 10-minute occlusions [29]. Rat myocardium has been successfully preconditioned with a single 5-minute occlusion in one study [30], while another group reported a single 5-minute occlusion was insufficient [31]. Multiple occlusion protocols in the rat have reported successful preconditioning following three 3-minute or three 5-minute occlusions [31,32], while three 2-minute occlusions reportedly have a borderline effect [33]. In addition to complete coronary occlusions, Ovize et al. [34] have shown that cyclic coronary flow variations, which result from formation and dislodgement of platelet-fibrin thrombi in denuded, constricted arteries, are also capable of inducing preconditioning. The same group also demonstrated that partial coronary stenosis without cyclic flow variations can trigger preconditioning [35].

A recent study by Shizukuda et al. [36] demonstrated that preconditioning could also be induced by hypoxia. These investigators created a 5-minute period of high-flow myocardial hypoxia by perfusing venous blood through a carotid-coronary conduit. The hypoxic episode was separated from a 60-minute sustained ischemic episode by a 10-minute period of normoxic perfusion. Infarct size in hypoxic-preconditioned animals was indistinguishable from that in animals that received a conventional 5-minute period of ischemia for preconditioning; both groups had infarcts markedly smaller than those of the control group. Interestingly, contractile function after the 60-minute occlusion was better in the hypoxic-preconditioned group compared to either the ischemic-preconditioned or control groups.

Perhaps the most surprising protocol reported to cause preconditioning was done by Przyklenk et al. [37]. These investigators performed four 5-minute occlusions of a branch of the *circumflex* artery, and after a 5-minute reperfusion period occluded the *left anterior descending coronary* for a 60-minute sustained ischemic episode. They reported that preconditioning the circumflex vascular bed protected the left anterior descending coronary vascular bed. The mechanism for this "preconditioning at a distance" is unknown, but could result from circulating ischemic metabolites, neuronal modulation, signalling via gap junctions, or mechanical dilation. As discussed above, it is also possible that this mechanism differs from that of more traditional preconditioning protocols.

It now seems likely that preconditioning is not an artifact restricted to the research laboratory. Importantly, Deutsch et al. [38] have provided evidence that preconditioning may occur in humans with coronary artery disease. These investigators studied patients undergoing two sequential 90-second balloon angioplasties of the left anterior descending coronary artery. The second episode of ischemia caused less chest pain, less ST-segment elevation, and less myocardial lactate production than the first. These changes were associated with reduced blood flow from the accompanying cardiac vein during the second occlusion. This suggests that the apparently less severe ischemia was not due to increased collateral blood flow, but rather reflected an adaptation of the myocardium to ischemia.

If preconditioning truly occurs in humans, it is possible that preinfarction ischemia (e.g., manifest as angina pectoris) might make the human heart more tolerant to a sustained occlusion and thereby slow the transmural progression of necrosis after complete coronary thrombosis. Several clinical studies of myocardial infarction have addressed this question either directly or indirectly, and unfortunately, there is no clear consensus. These studies are reviewed in detail in Chapter 10, and hence we shall not discuss them individually here. Two points regarding human studies of preconditioning and infarction, however, merit emphasis. First, based on our experimental observations that protection is lost when occlusions are maintained beyond a critical length (60–90 minutes in the dog), it seems logical that *human studies must have reperfusion therapy* if preconditioning is to be observed. Secondly, it is useful to consider the question, in which patients would we *not* expect preconditioning to occur? As discussed above, preconditioning can be induced experimentally by repeated total occlusion, intermittent thrombosis and thrombolysis, as well as by a fixed stenosis that induces only moderate ischemia. We speculate that these scenarios may encompass many (perhaps the majority?) of patients experiencing myocardial infarction. It could therefore be difficult to find a control group in which there was no ischemia preceding the onset of total occlusion. Although there are no data to support or refute this possibility, it could confound clinical attempts to study preconditioning.

LIMITS OF PROTECTION DURING SUSTAINED ISCHEMIA

Although dramatically protective during a 40-minute occlusion, we determined that preconditioning's protective effect was lost when the duration of the sustained occlusion was extended to 3 hours [3]. Subsequent studies have resolved this window of protection further. There is general agreement that infarct size is limited after a 60-minute occlusion [25], whereas after a 90-minute occlusion in dogs one study has reported protection [39], while another has shown no benefit [40]. Thus, although its effects in the early phase of ischemia are impressive, preconditioning is progressively less effective as the sustained occlusion is extended beyond 60 minutes in dogs.

From a theoretical standpoint the loss of protection could result from several possibilities. First, preconditioning could affect the subendocardial myocardium but not the subepicardial myocardium. We have direct evidence that this is not true, since the metabolic effects of preconditioning are seen in both the subendocardium and subepicardium (Murry, Reimer, and Jennings, unpublished observations). A second possibility is that preconditioning delays lethal injury only by a relatively short time, say, 15–20 minutes, and therefore makes a large difference when cell death is occurring rapidly (as in the subendocardium) but is much less impressive when cell death is slow (as in the subepicardium). This may be true. Cell death begins in the subendocardium at around 20 minutes, and by 40–60 minutes of ischemia a confluent subendocardial infarct will develop. In this case delaying the onset of lethal injury by 15 minutes would, in essence, convert a 40-minute occlusion into a 25-minute equivalent, scarcely into the lethal phase. On the other hand, cell death in the subepicardium begins between 60 and 90 minutes of ischemia and is completed between 3 and 6 hours. A 15-minute delay in an occlusion of this duration would be hard to detect (e.g., 75 vs. 90 minutes or 165 vs. 180 minutes). The fact that preconditioning does not limit infarct size after 90 minutes to 3 hours of ischemia may limit its direct clinical impact, since most patients do not seek (or receive) medical attention until after 3 hours of symptoms.

PROTECTION DECAYS WITH EXTENDED PERIODS OF INTERVENING REPERFUSION

If the time between preconditioning and the subsequent sustained occlusion is prolonged, the protective effect is gradually lost. The time course of preconditioning's decay, however, has not been characterized in a detailed fashion. In the dog (Figure 2), we showed that a single 15-minute preconditioning occlusion resulted in a dramatic infarct size limitation with only 5 minutes of intervening reperfusion (infarct size averaged 8% of that seen in the control group). When the intervening reperfusion was extended to 120 minutes, pre-

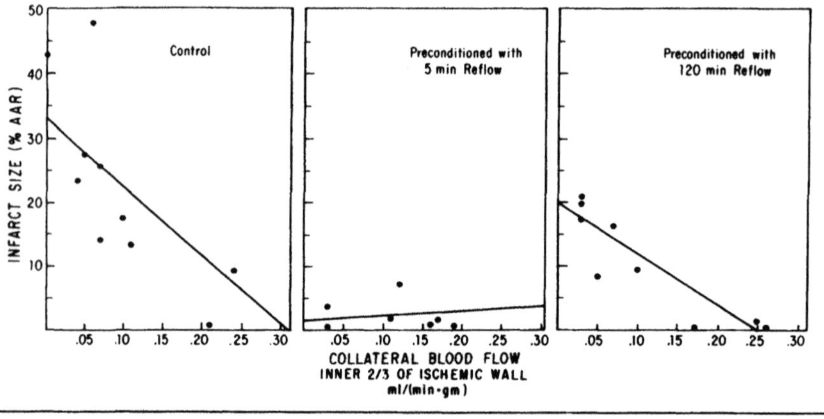

Figure 2. Effect of extending the intervening reperfusion period between preconditioning and the subsequent, sustained ischemic episode in dogs. Preconditioning was achieved by a single 15-minute occlusion of the left anterior descending coronary artery, which was separated from a 40-minute sustained test occlusion by either 5 minutes or 2 hours of intervening reperfusion. Control animals received a single 40-minute occlusion. Infarcts were sized histologically after 4 days of reperfusion and related to the anatomic area at risk and collateral blood flow, measured with radioactive microspheres administered midway through the sustained occlusion. In control hearts there was a general inverse relationship between infarct size and collateral blood flow, i.e., hearts with low collateral flow had large infarcts and vice versa. In the preconditioned group with 5 minutes of intervening reperfusion, infarcts were smaller than controls at any level of collateral blood flow ($p < 0.01$ by analysis of covariance). In the preconditioned group with 2 hours of intervening reperfusion, the regression line was intermediate between that of the control and the 5-minute reperfusion groups ($p < 0.05$ vs. control; $p < 0.01$ vs. 5-minute reflow group). This indicates that extending the length of reperfusion between preconditioning and sustained occlusion to 2 hours significantly attenuated preconditioning's protective effect. Reproduced from Murry et al. [26], by permission.

conditioning's protective effects were markedly attenuated (infarcts averaged 46% of control) [26]. In the rat, the effects of preconditioning with three 3-minute coronary occlusions were largely lost when the period of intervening reperfusion was extended from 5 minutes to 1 hour [32]. Miura et al. [41], using a single 5-minute preconditioning occlusion in rabbits, have recently reported significant loss of protection after only 25–35 minutes of intervening reperfusion. On the other hand, Schott et al. [29] reported marked protection in a pig model when 30 minutes of intervening reperfusion followed two 10-minute occlusions. Thus, the time course for the decay of ischemic tolerance may vary depending on the species and the particular protocol used to induce it. Within a given species, preconditioning protocols that cause more severe reversible injury may protect the myocardium for longer periods of ischemia, or their effects may decay more slowly during reperfusion; however, to our knowledge this has not been tested.

CHANGES IN MYOCARDIAL GENE EXPRESSION AND DELAYED PROTECTION: A SECOND WINDOW?

Brief episodes of ischemia induce changes in myocardial gene expression, including expression of protooncogenes and transcription factors, which are manifest within 1–3 hours [42], as well as expression of heat shock proteins [43], which become manifest 3–24 hours after the initial insult. Given this time delay, it is possible that a second window of protection could develop after the acute effects of preconditioning have waned. A recent study by Marber and colleagues [44] tested this hypothesis by subjecting rabbits to four 5-minute coronary occlusions, and then performing a 30-minute sustained test occlusion 24 hours later. Infarct size was significantly smaller in rabbits subjected to prior repeated ischemia than in sham-treated controls. A similar conclusion was reached in the preliminary report of Hoshida et al. [39], who used four 5-minute coronary occlusions to precondition dog hearts prior to a sustained occlusion of 90 minutes. They reported limitation of infarct size when the 90-minute occlusion immediately followed preconditioning. Protection was lost when the test occlusion was performed 3 or 6 hours after preconditioning, similar to our previous observations [26]. When the 90-minute occlusion was performed 24 hours after preconditioning, infarcts were again markedly smaller than controls.

The concept of a second window of cardioprotection, however, is controversial. Opposing these results is a study by Tanaka and Fujiwara [45], in which either one or four 5-minute occlusions were used to precondition rabbit hearts before a sustained 30-minute occlusion. Although infarcts were markedly smaller when the sustained occlusion was done within 5 minutes of preconditioning, no limitation of infarct size was observed after 2 or 24 hours of intervening reperfusion. Similarly, Donnelly et al. [46] failed to obtain a reduction in infarct size in rats subjected to brief ischemia 8 hours before the sustained period of ischemia. It is not clear why the studies disagree, particularly when the study by Tanaka and Fujiwara followed an almost identical protocol as the study by Marber and colleagues. The possibility of a second window of protection is a very important area for future research, one that could have direct implications for patients with coronary artery disease.

DOES ISCHEMIC PRECONDITIONING OCCUR OUTSIDE THE HEART?

In the remaining pages we shall review the available literature regarding the effects of multiple ischemic episodes in other organs. It will be useful to determine if preconditioning is a general reaction of cells to ischemic injury or if there are features unique to the myocardium that enable only the heart to mount this adaptive response. For example, preconditioning could be an adaptation unique to contractile cells, electrically excitable cells, cells with high capacity for aerobic metabolism or preference for certain metabolic substrates, or tissues with a rich autonomic innervation. By studying the phenomenon in other tissues we may derive clues to its mechanism in the heart.

Does preconditioning occur in the brain?

After the heart, the effects of repetitive, brief episodes of ischemia have been studied most extensively in the brain. To our knowledge the first studies were conducted by Tomida et al. [47]. These investigators utilized anesthetized gerbils and compared the effects of three 5-minute bilateral carotid occlusions with single 5- or 15-minute occlusions, all followed by 24 hours of reperfusion. In this model a single 5-minute occlusion caused only focal neuronal necrosis in the CA1 region of the hippocampus (the region most susceptible to ischemia), while a 15-minute occlusion caused more widespread hippocampal injury, as well as injury to the cortex. Surprisingly, the effects of three 5-minute occlusions varied widely, depending on the duration of intermittent reperfusion. If occlusions were separated by only 3 minutes of reperfusion, the injury was relatively mild, less extensive than seen after a single 15-minute occlusion. On the other hand, if the three 5-minute occlusions were each separated by 1 hour of intervening reperfusion, the injury was much more widespread than after a single 15-minute occlusion.

It is difficult to extrapolate from the previous study to our studies in the heart, because these authors used multiple occlusions that *individually* caused some cell death. Subsequently, however, Kato et al. studied the effects of repeated *reversible* ischemic insults in gerbils [48]. They reported that a single 2-minute occlusion caused no cell death, while three or five 2-minute occlusions, separated by 60 minutes of reperfusion, caused extensive cell death in multiple regions of the brain. Taken together, these studies indicate that the heart and brain react quite differently to repeated ischemic insults. Although multiple brief episodes of ischemia do not have a cumulative effect in the heart, they do in the brain and may even result in widespread necrosis. The reason for this difference is unknown. It is possible that repeated ischemic insults cause progressive brain edema, which, due to enclosure within a rigid calvarium, compresses the vasculature and prevents reflow. Tomida et al. [47] reported greater brain edema in animals receiving three 5-minute occlusions at 60-minute intervals. Whether this is cause or effect, however, is unclear.

Subsequent studies have directly addressed the ability of a brief episode of ischemia to protect the brain from an ensuing, longer ischemic insult. Kato et al. [49] performed a 2-minute bilateral carotid occlusion at varying intervals before a 3-minute occlusion. A single 2-minute occlusion caused no cell death, while a single 3-minute occlusion caused moderate necrosis of hippocampal CA1 neurons. When the two ischemic episodes were separated by 5 minutes to 6 hours of reperfusion there was *cumulative* injury, characterized by more widespread hippocampal necrosis. Intriguingly, when the ischemic episodes were separated by much longer reperfusion periods of 1–7 days, there was virtually no cell death. Protection was lost when the intervening reperfusion period was extended to 2 weeks. This effect also has been demonstrated in rats. Liu et al. [50] showed that a 3-minute episode of forebrain ischemia, followed by 3 days of reperfusion, was protective against subsequent ischemic episodes of 6 or 8 minutes, but was lost after a 10-minute sustained ischemic episode. They also demonstrated that a single 3-minute occlusion markedly increased immunohistochemical staining for heat shock protein 70 after 3 days of reperfusion.

Based on these experiments it seems clear that preconditioning, as originally defined for the heart, does not occur in brain. In short-term experiments, repeated occlusions have a cumulative deleterious effect. The protective effect seen between 1 and 7 days after a brief ischemic event, although termed *preconditioning* by Liu et al. [50], is almost certainly a different phenomenon from the acute adaptation we termed *myocardial preconditioning*. The duration required suggests that alterations in gene expression may play a role, and therefore this response in the brain may be similar to heat shock and other stress responses seen in the heart over a similar time frame [5].

Kidney, liver, and skeletal muscle

To our knowledge, only a few studies have addressed the response of other organs to repeated ischemic events. Zager et al. [51] studied the effects of an antecedent 15-minute renal artery occlusion on renal function, adenine nucleotides, and histology following a 25-minute occlusion. They reported that when the two occlusions were separated by 30 minutes of intervening reperfusion, renal function was worse (decreased glomerular filtration, increased serum creatinine and blood urea nitrogen), ATP depletion was more severe, and there was more tubular necrosis compared to controls receiving only a single 25-minute occlusion. No effect of the 15-minute occlusion was seen when the period of intervening reperfusion was extended to 3.5 or 24 hours. A subsequent study [52] reported that two intermittent reperfusion periods of 1.5 minutes did not preserve renal ATP levels after a cumulative 35-minute ischemic episode. Thus, although alternative multiple occlusion protocols should be explored (particularly using shorter occlusions), current evidence does not suggest preconditioning occurs in the kidney.

Isozaki et al. [53] compared the effects of continuous vs. intermittent ischemia in the rat liver. The portal vein and hepatic artery were occluded for total ischemic durations of 60, 90, or 120 minutes, and sustained ischemia was compared to multiple 15- or 30-minute occlusions with 5-minute reperfusion periods. After 60 minutes of total ischemia, when little injury had occurred, there was no benefit to intermittent reperfusion. After 90 and 120 minutes, however, intermittent reperfusion resulted in less hepatic transaminase enzyme release and fewer deaths compared to the sustained ischemia group; the two intermittent reperfusion groups were equivalent. These data are consistent with the beneficial effects of intermittent reperfusion in the heart, and we think a direct test of preconditioning in the liver would be worthwhile.

Finally, there is preliminary evidence that preconditioning occurs in skeletal muscle. Mounsey et al. [54] reported that a 30-minute ischemic episode reduced the necrosis by 20% in porcine latissimus dorsi muscles after a sustained 4-hour occlusion. Given the structural and biochemical similarities between skeletal and cardiac muscle, this would not be unexpected. The small group size (n = 5) precludes definitive conclusion, however.

SUMMARY AND FUTURE DIRECTIONS

Since our initial report of the phenomenon in 1986 there has been explosive growth in our understanding of preconditioning's effects on the heart and its underlying mechanisms. Much of this new information is summarized in subsequent chapters of this book. If we are to extend preconditioning's protective effects to patients by drug therapy, it will be necessary to understand the mechanism through which it works, particularly the signalling pathways that lead to myocyte responses. From the experimentalist's standpoint, preconditioning represents an opportunity to learn much about the pathogenesis of lethal ischemic injury, particularly the late events that influence the proximate causes of cell death. Finally, the fact that brief ischemic episodes induce short- and long-term changes in signalling pathways, metabolism, and gene expression tells us that the myocardium of patients with chronic ischemic heart disease may be much different than we originally imagined. Understanding these adaptive changes may eventually lead to improved therapy for the ischemic heart.

REFERENCES

1. Reimer KA, Jennings RB, Tatum AH. 1983. Pathobiology of acute myocardial ischemia: Metabolic, functional and ultrastructural studies. Am J Cardiol 52:72A–81A.
2. Hearse DJ, Yellon DM. 1984. Why are we still in doubt about infarct size limitation?

The experimentalist's viewpoint. In Therapeutic Approaches to Myocardial Infarct Size Limitation, DJ Hearse, DM Yellon, eds. Raven Press, New York, pp. 17–41.

3. Murry CE, Jennings RB, Reimer KA. 1986. preconditioning with ischemia: A delay of lethal cell injury in ischemic myocardium. Circulation 74:1124–1136.
4. Schott RJ, Nao B, Strieter R, Groh M, Kunkel S, McClanahan T, Schaper W, Gallagher K. 1990. Heat shock does not "precondition" canine myocardium. Circulation 82(Suppl III): III464 (abstr).
5. Yellon DM, Latchman DS. 1992. Stress proteins and myocardial protection. J Mol Cell Cardiol 24:113–124.
6. Liu G, Downey JM. 1992. Acetylcholine preconditions rabbit heart: Further evidence for Gi protein coupling in preconditioning. Circulation 86(Suppl I):I174 (abstr).
7. Ovize M, Przyklenk K, Kloner RA. 1992. Myocardial dilation, in the absence of ischemia, preconditions the canine heart. Circulation 86(Suppl I):I32 (abstr).
8. Shiki K, Hearse DJ. 1987. Preconditioning of ischemic myocardium: Reperfusion-induced arrhythmias. Am J Physiol 253:H1470–H1476.
9. Hagar JM, Hale SL, Kloner RA. 1991. Effect of preconditioning ischemia on reperfusion arrhythmias after coronary artery occlusion and reperfusion in the rat. Circ Res 68:61–68.
10. Urabe K, Miura T, Iwamoto T, Ogawa T, Endoh A, Iimura O. 1992. Preconditioning attenuates myocardial stunning via adenosine receptor activation. Circulation 86(Suppl I):I24 (abstr).
11. Miyazaki T, Zipes DP. 1989. Protection against autonomic denervation following acute myocardial infarction by preconditioning ischemia. Circ Res 64:437–448.
12. DeFily DV, Chilian WM. 1991. Preconditioning protects coronary microvascular endothelial function. Circulation 84(Suppl II):II434 (abstr).
13. Jennings RB, Hawkins HD, Lowe JE, Hill ML, Klotman S, Reimer KA. 1978. Relation between high energy phosphate and lethal injury in myocardial ischemia in the dog. Am J Pathol 92:187–214.
14. Neely JR, Grotyohann LW. 1984. Role of glycolytic products in damage to ischemic myocardium. Dissociation of adenosine triphosphate levels and recovery of function of reperfused ischemic hearts. Circ Res 55:816–824.
15. Swain JL, Sabina RL, McHale PA, Greenfield JC, Jr., Holmes EW. 1982. Prolonged myocardial adenine nucleotide depletion after brief ischemia in the open-chest dog. Am J Physiol 242:H818–H826.
16. Reimer KA, Hill ML, Jennings RB. 1981. Prolonged depletion of ATP and of the adenine nucleotide pool due to delayed resynthesis of adenine nucleotides following reversible myocardial ischemic injury in dogs. J Mol Cell Cardiol 13:229–239.
17. DeBoer LWV, Ingwall JS, Kloner RA, Braunwald E. 1980. Prolonged derangements of canine myocardial purine metabolism after a brief coronary artery occlusion not associated with anatomic evidence of necrosis. Proc Natl Acad Sci USA 77:5471–5475.
18. Reimer KA, Murry CE, Yamasawa I, Hill ML, Jennings RB. 1986. Four brief periods of ischemia cause no cumulative ATP loss or necrosis. Am J Physiol 251:H1306–H1315.
19. Lange R, Ingwall JS, Hale SL, Alker KJ, Kloner RA. 1984. Effects of recurrent ischemia on myocardial high energy phosphate content in canine hearts. Basic Res Cardiol 79:469–478.
20. Hoffmeister HM, Mauser M, Schaper W. 1986. Repeated short periods of regional myocardial ischemia: Effect on local function and high energy phosphate levels. Basic Res Cardiol 81:361–372.
21. Swain JL, Sabina RL, Hines JJ, Greenfield JC, Jr., Holmes EW. 1984. Repetitive episodes of brief ischaemia (12 min) do not produce a cumulative depletion of high energy phosphate compounds. Cardiovasc Res 18:264–269.
22. Henrichs KJ, Matsuoka H, Schaper J. 1987. Influence of repetitive coronary occlusions on myocardial adenine nucleosides, high energy phosphates and ultrastructure. Basic Res Cardiol 82:557–565.
23. Jennings RB, Schaper J, Hill ML, Steenbergen C, Reimer KA. 1985. Effect of repefusion late in the phase of reversible ischemic injury. Changes in cell volume, electrolytes, metabolites and ultrastructure. Circ Res 56:262–278.
24. Ovize M, Przyklenk K, Hale SL, Kloner RA. 1992. Preconditioning does not attenuate myocardial stunning. Circulation 85:2247–2254.
25. Li GC, Vasquez JA, Gallagher KP, Lucchesi BR. 1990. Myocardial protection with precon-

ditioning. Circuklation 82:609–619.
26. Murry CE, Richard VJ, Jennings RB, Reimer KA. 1991. Myocardial protection is lost before contractile function recovers from ischemic preconditioning. Am J Physiol 260: H796–H804.
27. Miura T, Noto T, Adachi T, Endoh A, Goto M, Urabe K, Iimura O. 1990. Does myocardial stunning contribute to infarct limitation by preconditioning? Circulation 82(Suppl III):40 (abstr).
28. Liu GS, Thornton J, Van Winkle DM, Stanley AWH, Olsson RA, Downey JM. 1991. Protection against infarction afforded by preconditioning is mediated by A1 adenosine receptors in the rabbit heart. Circulation 84:350–356.
29. Schott RJ, Rohmann S, Braun ER, Schapter W. 1990. Ischemic preconditioning reduces infarct size in swine myocardium. Circ Res 66:1133–1142.
30. Yellon DM, Alkhulaifi AM, Browne EE, Pugsley WB. 1992. Ischaemic preconditioning limits infarct size in the rat heart. Cardiovasc Res 26:983–987.
31. Liu Y, Downey JM. 1992. Ischemic preconditioning protects against infarction in rat heart. Am J Physiol 263:H1107–1112.
32. Li Y, Whittaker P, Kloner RA. 1992. The transient nature of the effect of ischemic preconditioning on myocardial infarct size and ventricular arrhythmia. Am Heart J 123:346–353.
33. Matsuoka H, Terui G, Kimura H, Hasegawa H, Ueki K, Kibira S, Miura M. 1992. Role of adenosine in ischemic preconditioning in rat heart. Circulation 86(Suppl I):I24 (abstr).
34. Ovize M, Kloner RA, Hale SL, Przyklenk K. 1992. Coronary cyclic flow variations "precondition" ischemic myocardium. Circulation 85:779–789.
35. Ovize M, Przyklenk K, Kloner RA. 1992. Partial coronary stenosis is sufficient and complete reperfusion is mandatory for preconditioning in the canine heart. Circ Res 71: 1165–1173.
36. Shizukuda Y, Mallet RT, Lee S-C, Downey HF. 1992. Hypoxic preconditioning of ischaemic canine myocardium. Cardiovasc Res 26:534–542.
37. Przyklenk K, Bauer B, Ovize M, Kloner RA, Whittaker P. 1993. Regional ischemic "preconditioning" protects remote virgin myocardium from subsequent sustained coronary occlusion. Circulation 87:839–899.
38. Deutsch E, Berger M, Kussmaul WG, Hirshfeld JW, Jr, Herrmann HC, Laskey WK. 1990. Adaptation to ischemia during percutaneous transluminal coronary angioplasty: Clinical, hemodynamic, and metabolic features. Circulation 82:2044–2051.
39. Hoshida S, Kuzuya T, Yamashita N, Fuji H, Oe H, Otsu K, Kimura Y, Hori M, Tada M. 1992. Delayed effect of sublethal ischemia on limiting infarct size resulting from sustained ischemia and reperfusion. Circulation 86(Suppl I):I30 (abstr).
40. Nao BS, McClanahan TB, Groh MA, Schott RJ, Gallagher KP. 1990. The time limit of effective ischemic preconditioning in dogs. Circulation 82(Suppl III):271 (abstr).
41. Miura T, Adachi T, Ogawa T, Iwamoto T, Tsuchida A, Iimura O. 1992. Myocardial infarct size-limiting effect of ischemic preconditioning: Its natural decay and the effect of repetitive preconditioning. Cardiovasc Pathol 1:147–154.
42. Brand T, Sharma HS, Fleischmann KE, Duncker DJ, McFalls EO, Verdouw PD, Schaper W. 1992. Proto-oncogene expression in porcine myocardium subjected to ischemia and reperfusion. Circ Res 71:1351–1360.
43. Knowlton AA, Brecher P, Ngoy S, Apstein CS. 1991. Rapid expression of heat shock protein in the rabbit after brief cardiac ischemia. J Clin Invest 87:139–147.
44. Marber MS, Latchman DS, Walker JM, Yellon DM. 1993. Cardiac stress protein elevation 24 hours following brief ischemia or heat stress is associated with resistance to myocardial infarction. Circulation, in press.
45. Tanaka M, Fujiwara H. 1992. Is the time course of infarct size limiting effect of ischemic preconditioning bimodal? Circulation 86(Suppl I):I34 (abstr).
46. Donnelly TJ, Sievers RE, Vissern FLJ, Welch WJ, Wolfe CL. 1992. Heat shock protein induction in rats: A role for improved myocardial salvage after ischemia and reperfusion? Circulation 85:769–778.
47. Tomida S, Nowak TS, Jr., Vass K, Lohr JM, Klatzo I. 1987. Experimental model for repetitive ischemic attacks in the gerbil: The cumulative effect of repeated ischemic insults. J Cereb Blood Flow Metab 7:773–782.
48. Kato H, Kogure K, Nakano S. 1989. Neuronal damage following repeated brief ischemia in the gerbil. Brain Res 479:366–370.

49. Kato H, Liu Y, Araki T, Kogure K. 1991. Temporal profile of the effects of pretreatment with brief cerebral ischemia on the neuronal damage following secondary ischemic insult in the gerbil: Cumulative damage and protective effects. Brain Res 553:238–242.
50. Liu Y, Kato H, Nakata N, Kogure K. 1992. Protection of rat hippocampus against ischemic neuronal damage by pretreatment with sublethal ischemia. Brain Res 586:121–124.
51. Zager RA, Jurkowitz MS, Merola AJ. 1985. Responses of the normal rat kidney to sequential ischemic events. Am J Physiol 249:F148–F159.
52. Thornton MA, Zager RA. 1990. Brief intermittent reperfusion during renal ischemia: Effects on adenine nucleotides, oxidant stress, and the severity of renal failure. J Lab Clin Med 115:564–571.
53. Isozaki H, Adam R, Gigou M, Szekely AM, Shen M, Bismuth H. 1992. Experimental study of the protective effect of intermittent hepatic pedicle clamping in the rat. Br J Surg 79:310–313.
54. Mounsey RA, Pang CY, Forrest C. 1992. Preconditioning: A new technique for improved muscle flap survival. Otolaryngol Head Neck Surg 107:549–552.

2. PRECONDITIONING AND ISCHEMIA- AND REPERFUSION-INDUCED ARRHYTHMIAS

CLIVE S. LAWSON and DAVID J. HEARSE

HISTORY OF PRECONDITIONING AND ARRHYTHMOGENESIS

The term *preconditioning* is currently employed primarily to describe the enhanced resistance to ischemia-induced myocardial necrosis afforded by one or more brief preceding episodes of ischemia and reperfusion. Indeed, some investigators believe that the term should be reserved strictly for studies where myocardial protection is expressed as a limitation of myocardial infarct size. Quite why such a limited usage should be suggested is, in our opinion, not clear. Historically, of course, the term *preconditioning with ischemia* was first coined in the context of infarct size limitation in dogs [1]. That report, and the many subsequent confirmations of the potency of preconditioning (for review, see reference [2]), generated a great deal of excitement, principally because, with the exception of reperfusion, no previous intervention had proven able to afford a sustained limitation of infarct size under carefully controlled experimental conditions. Myocardial protection, however, can be manifest in a number of different ways, and the study by Murry et al. [1] was by no means the first to document altered myocardial responses to serial challenges. Two years earlier Neely and Grotyhan [3] had described the protective effect of a period of hypoxic perfusion on contractile dysfunction and the accumulation of metabolic products following an ischemic challenge. The first indications of the antiarrhythmic properties of what might now be considered ischemic preconditioning, however, were published even earlier [4] and predate Murry's classical paper [1] by more than 30 years.

In 1950 Harris [4] described the use of a two-stage coronary ligation procedure, partial occlusion prior to total occlusion, which led to a dramatic reduction in the number of early ischemia-induced ventricular premature beats (VPBs). In 1977 Gulker el al. [5] reported that repeated episodes of ischemia and reperfusion were associated with an increase in the threshold for the precipitation of ventricular fibrillation (VF) by programmed electrical stimulation in dogs. Subsequently Barber [6] reported that serial 5-minute coronary occlusions led to reductions in both the extent of ST-segment elevation and the number of ischemia-induced VPBs. These results were met with rather limited acclaim, presumably because there were many preceding reports of effective antiarrhythmic interventions and also because the degree of protection was not particularly profound. Nevertheless, as the initial descriptions of the protective effects of brief episodes of ischemia and reperfusion were recorded in studies employing arrhythmias as their principal end point, on historical grounds alone it would appear inappropriate to limit the term *preconditioning* to protection against myocardial necrosis. Indeed, subsequent studies have demonstrated that preconditioning can, in some models, afford very profound protection against both ischemia- and reperfusion-induced arrhythmias. It remains to be determined, however, if antiarrhythmic protection is a direct consequence of antiischemic protection and if the molecular mechanisms involved are the same as those involved in protection against necrosis.

PRECONDITIONING AND REPERFUSION-INDUCED ARRHYTHMIAS

Can preconditioning prevent malignant arrhythmias?

Shiki and Hearse [7] were the first to show that preconditioning could actually prevent *malignant* arrhythmias. They examined its effect on the severity of reperfusion-induced arrhythmias in rat hearts in vivo using paired coronary occlusions separated by a variable time period. The severity of reperfusion-induced arrhythmias following the second ischemic episode was substantially reduced, with the abolition of reperfusion-induced VF and VPBs, a profound reduction in the incidence of reperfusion-induced ventricular tachycardia (VT), and an increase in the time-in-sinus-rhythm following reperfusion (Figure 1). Protection could be demonstrated provided that the first coronary occlusion lasted for at least 3 minutes and that the second challenge occurred within 1 hour of the first. The temporal aspects of this protection against reperfusion-induced arrhythmias are remarkably similar to those of protection against myocardial necrosis reported by others [1,8].

The study by Shiki and Hearse [7], however,provided a new insight into the rapidity of onset of preconditioning-induced protection. In studies where myocardial infarct size is assessed, an experimental duration of several hours

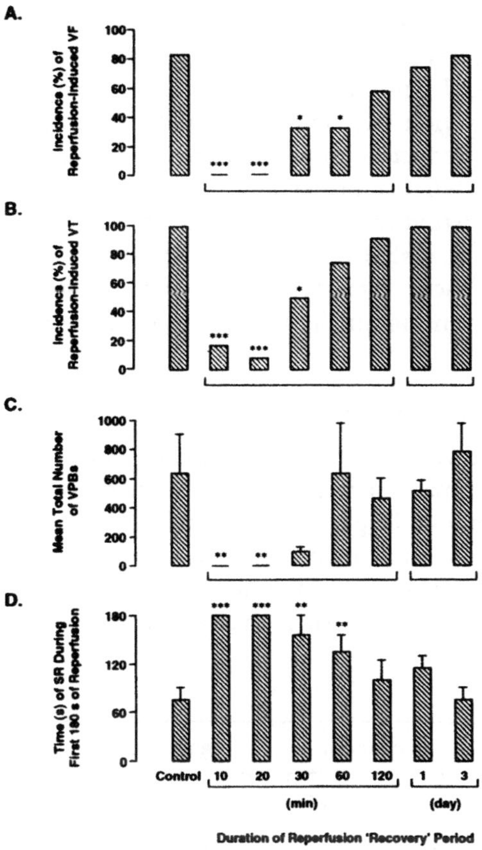

Figure 1. Relationship between duration of "recovery" and vulnerability of the heart to arrhythmias induced by reperfusion after a second episode (5 minutes) of regional ischemia in vivo. Hearts (n = 12 per group) were subjected to 5 minutes of regional ischemia followed by reperfusion for 10, 20, 30, 60, or 120 minutes or 3 days, after which regional ischemia was again induced for a period of 5 minutes. Histograms show the incidence of ventricular fibrillation (**A**), incidence of ventricular tachycardia (**B**), mean total number of ventricular premature complexes (**C**), and mean time in normal sinus rhythm during the first 3 minutes of reperfusion (**D**). Results are compared with control group, which corresponds to values obtained after the first period of ischemia and reperfusion. * $p < 0.05$, ** $p < 0.01$, *** $p < 0.0001$ vs. control group. Reproduced with permission from Shiki and Hearse [7].

is required before the extent of necrosis can be accurately quantified. Under these circumstances it is not possible to determine how quickly protection is manifest. Protection against reperfusion-induced arrhythmias, however, was demonstrated within 15 minutes of the first coronary occlusion, indicating that whatever adaptive physiological process underlies this protection, it must occur very rapidly.

A further important finding of the above study was that the protection against arrhythmias following the second challenge was in direct proportion to the severity of the arrhythmias precipitated by the first. This raised the possibility that hearts have a "quota" of arrhythmias that, once precipitated, cannot be reinduced without an intervening recovery period. Although pertinent, this observation may explain in part the reluctance of some investigators to accept a reduction of arrhythmia severity as a true manifestation of preconditioning-mediated protection. If such a quota did exist it would indicate that antiarrhythmic protection by preconditioning is *dependent* on the precipitation of arrhythmias by the preconditioning stimulus. From a practical point of view, there would appear to be little clinical benefit to be gained from "preventing" malignant arrhythmias by their precipitation at an earlier stage.

Is arrhythmia precipitation by preconditioning necessary?

It is now clear, however, that it is not essential for preconditioning protocols to induce arrhythmias themselves before antiarrhythmic protection can be subsequently manifest. Hagar et al. [9] performed an in vivo study in rats in which, in order to limit arrhythmia precipitation during preconditioning, they reduced the duration of individual episodes of preconditioning ischemia to 2 minutes. Using three such cycles, each separated by 5 minutes of

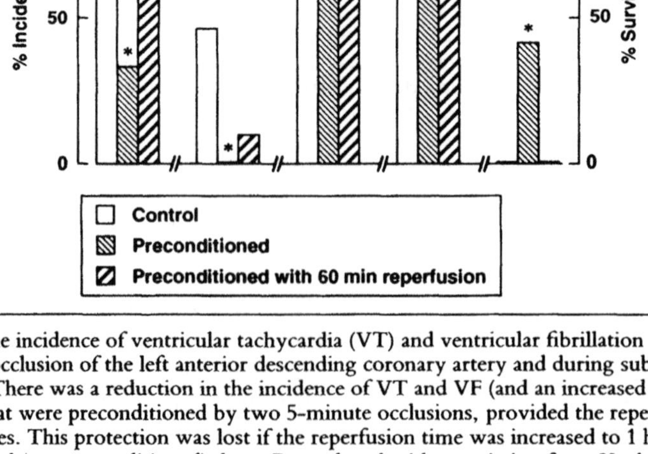

Figure 2. The incidence of ventricular tachycardia (VT) and ventricular fibrillation (VF) during a 25-minute occlusion of the left anterior descending coronary artery and during subsequent reperfusion. There was a reduction in the incidence of VT and VF (and an increased survival) in those dogs that were preconditioned by two 5-minute occlusions, provided the reperfusion time was 20 minutes. This protection was lost if the reperfusion time was increased to 1 hour. *$p < 0.05$ vs. control (nonpreconditioned) dogs. Reproduced with permission from Vegh et al. [10].

reperfusion, they were able to demonstrate substantial protection against reperfusion-induced arrhythmias, contrary to the concept of an "arrhythmia quota." Again VF was abolished and the incidence of VT reduced from 100% to 25%. Similarly, Vegh et al. [10] have since shown that protection against reperfusion-induced VF is possible in dogs without the precipitation of malignant arrhythmias during the preconditioning phase (Figure 2).

True protection or temporal shift of vulnerability?

A major limitation of all of these studies, however, is their restriction to the study of reperfusion-induced arrhythmias occurring following a single ischemic duration. The severity of reperfusion-induced arrhythmias is critically dependent on the duration of the preceding period of ischemia, and the relationship between the two is bell-shaped for dogs and rats [11]. Following very brief episodes of ischemia (i.e., less than 3 minutes), little ischemic damage occurs and the incidence of reperfusion-induced arrhythmias is low. Similarly, if the ischemic duration is very prolonged (i.e., more than 1 hour), irreversible injury occurs and reperfusion of nonviable myocardium does not lead to arrhythmia precipitation. Between these extremes (i.e., with ischemic durations of 5–20 minutes) the myocardium is highly vulnerable to the precipitation of malignant arrhythmias by reperfusion and high incidences occur.

Ischemic preconditioning could affect the bell-shaped relationship in three distinct ways. These are represented diagrammatically in Figure 3.

Rightward shift in time:vulnerability profile

Ischemic preconditioning classically delays the development of ischemia-induced myocardial necrosis [1]. If the beneficial action of preconditioning on reperfusion-induced arrhythmias occurs as a consequence of a similar increase in the ischemic tolerance, this would be expected to result in a shift in the bell-shaped curve to the right (Figure 3A).

Leftward shift in time:vulnerability profile

Conversely, serial ischemic episodes could lead to cumulative ischemic damage. This would be expected to shift the bell-shaped curve to the left but could still lead to a reduction in severity of reperfusion-induced arrhythmias being recorded, dependent on the duration of ischemia studied (Figure 3B). Osada et al. [12] demonstrated that preconditioning could reduce the incidence of reperfusion-induced arrhythmias following sequential 15-minute episodes of global ischemia in rats. Such a protocol might, however, produce cumulative ischemic damage and even produce irreversible myocardial injury. This study epitomizes the difficulty in being certain that a protective effect of preconditioning against reperfusion-induced arrhythmias represents a genuinely beneficial change when a single ischemic duration is employed.

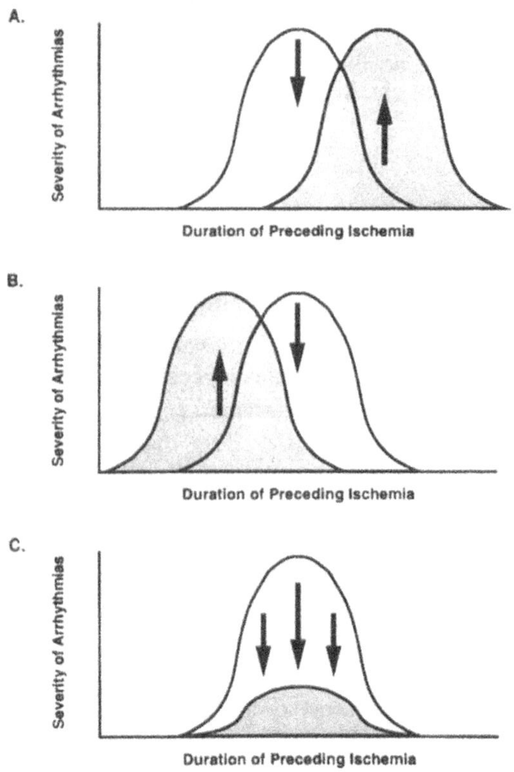

Figure 3. Schematic diagram of the possible effects of ischemic preconditioning on the bell-shaped relationship between the severity of reperfusion-induced arrhythmias and the duration of preceding ischemia. **A**: If preconditioning acts by increasing ischemic tolerance, a shift in the relationship to the right might be expected; dependent on the duration of preceding ischemia, either a reduction or an increase (arrows) in the severity of reperfusion-induced arrhythmias could be recorded. **B**: If cumulative ischemic damage occurred, a shift in the relationship to the left might be expected; again, dependent on the duration of preceding ischemia, either a reduction or an increase (arrows) in the severity of reperfusion-induced arrhythmias could be recorded. **C**: If preconditioning protects against arrhythmias as a consequence of an antiarrhythmic effect distinct from its antiischemic actions, this might be expected to result in a reduction to result in arrhythmia severity irrespective of the duration of ischemia studied (arrows).

Downward shift in time:vulnerability profile

With rightward or leftward shifts of the time-vulnerability profile, the effect on the measured severity of reperfusion-induced arrhythmias can be either an increase or a decrease, dependent on the ischemic duration studied. A third possibility, however, is that preconditioning might act to reduce the incidence of reperfusion-induced arrhythmias following all ischemic durations without altering the ischemic time associated with maximum severity of arrhythmias (i.e., without producing a temporal shift of the bell-shaped curve — Figure 3C).

Thus, an important consequence of the bell-shaped relationship is that, where only a single ischemic duration is studied, it is possible for repeated ischemic episodes to lead to a reduction in the severity of reperfusion-induced arrhythmias without the first episode *necessarily* having increased the ischemic tolerance of the myocardium. We have recently undertaken a study to determine which of these three possible effects preconditioning has on the bell-shaped relationship [13]. Using isolated rat hearts perfused with blood, we have induced ischemic preconditioning using three cycles of 5 minutes of regional ischemia and 5 minutes of reperfusion and assessed its effect on the severity of reperfusion-induced arrhythmias occurring following ischemic

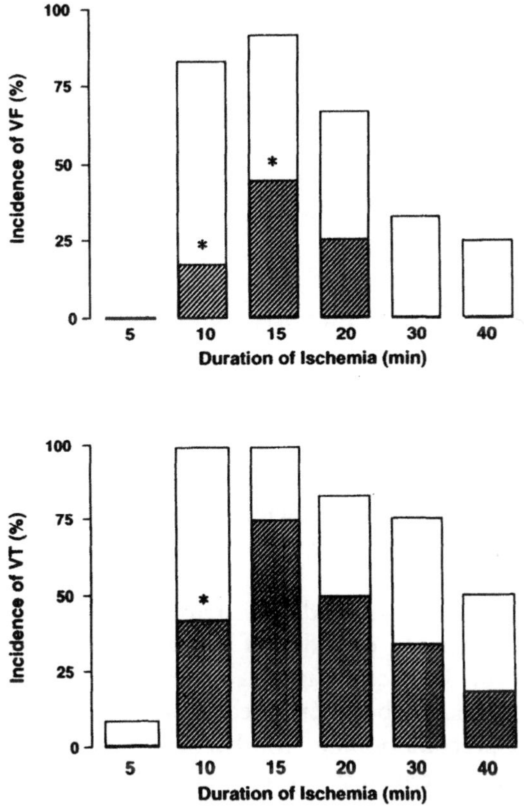

Figure 4. Effect of preconditioning on the bell-shaped relationship between the incidence of reperfusion-induced arrhythmias and the duration of preceding ischemia. The incidence of reperfusion-induced ventricular fibrillation (top) and ventricular tachycardia (bottom) is compared in control and preconditioned rat hearts following 5, 10, 15, 20, 30, or 40 minutes of ischemia (n = 12 per group). Open bars = control; hatched bars = preconditioned. VF, ventricular fibrillation; VT, ventricular tachycardia. *$p < 0.05$ vs. respective control group.

durations ranging from 5 to 40 minutes. For each ischemic duration studied there was a reduction in the severity of reperfusion-induced arrhythmias. In addition, the peak incidence of reperfusion-induced VT and VF occurred after 15 minutes of ischemia in both control and preconditioned hearts, indicating no temporal shift in the bell-shaped relationship (Figure 4). This result has important implications for the mechanism of preconditioning-mediated protection against reperfusion-induced arrhythmias: It suggests such protection is not primarily due to an alteration in ischemic tolerance, and indicates that preconditioning has an additional and distinct antiarrhythmic action.

PRECONDITIONING AND ISCHEMIA-INDUCED ARRHYTHMIAS

Does preconditioning protect against ischemia-induced arrhythmias?

When Murry et al. [1] first described the capacity of ischemic preconditioning to limit infarct size in dogs, they reported no protection against arrhythmias. Indeed, in subsequent studies the same group have reported an increase in arrhythmic mortality [14]. It is important to note, however, that many of these deaths occurred as a consequence of the preconditioning protocol rather than during the later prolonged ischemic episode. This is indicative, therefore, of a limitation of the preconditioning protocol employed in those studies, rather than of a lack of antiarrhythmic efficacy of preconditioning.

Vegh et al. [10,15] reported the first studies designed specifically to assess the effect of preconditioning in dogs using ischemia-induced arrhythmias as the primary end point. With two sequential 5-minute episodes of preconditioning ischemia, less than 15% of animals suffered sustained tachyarrhythmias as a consequence of preconditioning. The effect on the severity of arrhythmias during a subsequent prolonged ischemic episode, however, was profound. VF was abolished, the incidence of VT reduced from over 80% to less than 40% (Figure 2), and the mean number of VPBs reduced to 21% of the control level.

Protection against ischemia-induced arrhythmias has also been shown to occur following 2-minute episodes of demand ischemia induced by rapid pacing in dogs [16]. Protection against reperfusion-induced arhythmias was less marked. It remains to be determined to what extent this represents a true manifestation of preconditioning. Marber has reported that rapid pacing in rabbits does not protect against myocardial necrosis [17].

Reduction in severity or delay in onset?

As with reperfusion-induced arrhythmias, the question arises as to whether protection against ischemia-induced arrhythmias is a consequence of a true reduction in arrhythmia severity or simply a delaying effect such that the arrhythmias are not manifest during the ischemic period studied. As preconditioning delays myocardial necrosis, it might be expected that a delaying action on the temporal pattern of arrhythmias might be observed.

Most studies of preconditioning and ischemia-induced arrhythmias reported to date have concentrated on those that occur during the early phase of ischemia, which, dependent on species, typically peak in severity after 10–20 minutes and subside within 30–40 minutes after coronary occlusion. To distinguish between a true antiarrhythmic action and a delaying effect, it is essential that the ischemic duration should be sufficiently prolonged to ensure that delayed arrhythmias are not missed. The ischemic duration employed in the first study reported by Vegh et al. [15] was only 25 minutes and thus insufficient to allow such a distinction to be made. More recently, however, the same group have confirmed, in a small number of dogs, that even when the ischemic period is extended to 60 minutes there is no evidence of a delaying effect on VPBs [10].

The same appears to be true for rats. With an ischemic period of 90 minutes Li et al. [8] demonstrated, in the in vivo rat model, that the reduction in arrhythmia severity is a consequence of reduced arrhythmia incidence with no evidence of any delayed arrhythmias (Figure 5). However, these in vivo studies suffer from significant data censoring due to animal mortality as a consequence not only of arrhythmias but also hypotension. In one such study, for example, 50 of the 86 rats studied failed to complete the experimental protocol [8]. This raises the possibility that delayed arrhythmias

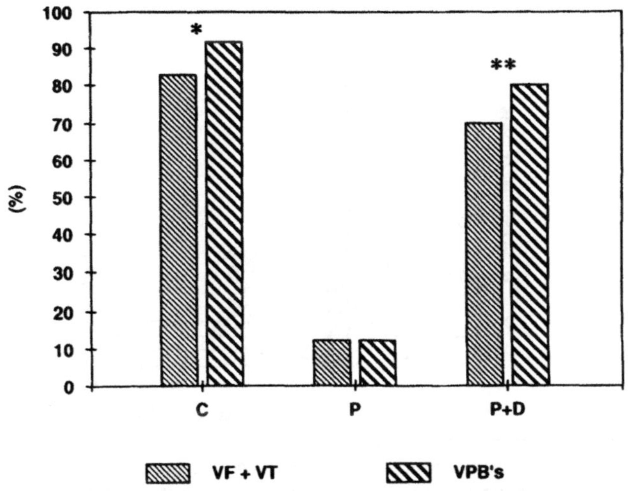

Figure 5. The effect of preconditioning on the incidence of arrhythmia (ventricular premature beats, ventricular tachycardia, or ventricular fibrillation) during the 90-minute period of occlusion. *p < 0.03 vs. preconditioning group by Fisher exact test (two-tail), P, Preconditioned group; P+D, preconditioned + delayed occlusion group (1-, 2-, and 3-hour delay); C, nonpreconditioned controls. Reproduced with permission from Li et al. [8].

would have occurred had the animal survived, but were not seen due to prior mortality from other causes. In addition, the antiarrhythmic effect of preconditioning in rats is so profound that very few malignant arrhythmias occur during ischemia in preconditioned hearts when a fully effective preconditioning protocol is employed, thus confounding a detailed analysis of their time course.

To resolve the issue of whether preconditioning abolishes or merely delays the development of ischemia-induced arrhythmias, we have performed a study in isolated rat hearts [18]. As the hearts are isolated from the hemodynamic consequences of arrhythmias, data censoring late in the protocol is limited. The results of this study are represented in Figure 6. During each

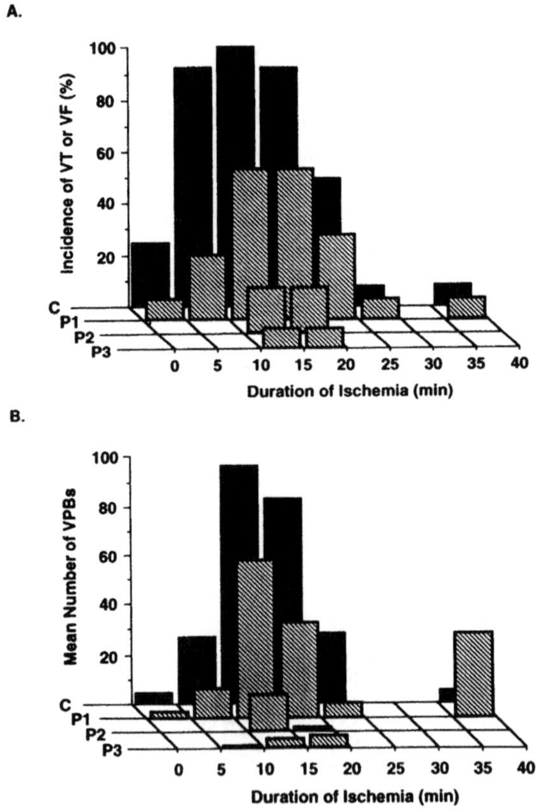

Figure 6. The effect of ischemic preconditioning on (**A**) the incidence of ventricular tachycardia or fibrillation and (**B**) the mean number of ventricular premature beats in isolated blood-perfused rat hearts assessed over sequential 5-minute time periods during a 40-minute ischemic episode. VF = ventricular fibrillation; VT = ventricular tachycardia; VPB = ventricular premature beats. Preconditioning induced by cycles of 5 minutes of ischemia and 5 minutes of reperfusion. Study groups (n = 12 per group); C = control, P1 = 1 preconditioning cycle, P2 = two preconditioning cycles, and P3 = three preconditioning cycles.

5-minute time band of a 40-minute ischemic period, preconditioning led to reductions in the incidences of sustained tachyarrhythmias (i.e., VF and VT) and VPBs; however, with this experimental preparation graded antiarrhythmic protection occurs with increasing numbers of preconditioning cycles. The use of two or three cycles of preconditioning ischemia led to the virtual abolition of ischemia-induced arrhythmias, but with a single cycle an intermediate degree of protection occurred. In all groups, however, the time of peak vulnerability to arrhythmias was between 10 and 20 minutes, and little arrhythmic activity occurred after 25 minutes of ischemia in any group. Thus, despite substantial protection, there was again no evidence of any significant temporal shift in the pattern of vulnerability to ischemia-induced arrhythmias, confirming that arrhythmias are abolished, rather than merely delayed, as a result of preconditioning. As with reperfusion-induced arrhythmias, this pattern is contrary to what might be expected if protection is a consequence of an increase in ischemic tolerance.

DOSE DEPENDENCY OF ANTIARRHYTHMIC PROTECTION

Using a single cycle of 3 minutes of preconditioning ischemia, Vegh et al. [10] were able to precondition effectively against ischemia-induced arrhythmias in rats hearts in vivo. They demonstrated reductions in the mean total duration of VT and the number of VPBs, but they did not show reductions in the *incidence* of either VF or VT. Conversely, when Li et al. [8] used three cycles of 3 minutes of ischemia to precondition rat hearts, they showed not only protection against VPBs but also marked reductions in the incidence of ischemia-induced VF and VT. The reduction in incidence of malignant arrhythmias following three preconditioning cycles in this study [8], in contrast to the less profound attenuation of their duration following a single cycle [10] in a virtually identical model, might indicate additional antiarrhythmic benefit from the second and third preconditioning cycles.

As shown in Figure 6, using isolated rat hearts perfused with blood, we have recently shown that protection against ischemia-induced arrhythmias is indeed cumulative with up to three cycles of preconditioning ischemia and reperfusion. A similar pattern of dose-dependent protection with up to three preconditioning cycles also occurs for reperfusion-induced arrhythmias in this model [19].

Most studies have indicated that for protection against myocardial necrosis a single preconditioning cycle is as effective as multiple cycles [20,21]. It is difficult to conceive, however, of a physiological process that might underlie preconditioning and possess such an all-or-nothing action. Rather surprisingly, Liu and Downey [22] have recently shown that in rat hearts in vivo, a single cycle of 5 minutes of ischemia is sufficient to virtually abolish ischemia-induced arrhythmias, but that three cycles are required before protection against myocardial necrosis can be demonstrated. Thus, dose dependency for preconditioning can be demonstrated under certain experimental conditions. It appears, however, that those conditions are different for necrosis and arrhythmias. Interestingly, at least in rats, preconditioning appears to be more potent in preventing arrhythmias than necrosis.

IS ANTIARRHYTHMIC PROTECTION SPECIES-DEPENDENT?

One of the most remarkable features of ischemic preconditioning has been the consistency of protection against myocardial necrosis reported by different laboratories. Indeed it has proven possible in all species studied to show a reduction in infarct size following preconditioning [2,23]. In contrast, the antiarrhythmic properties of preconditioning have been reported to occur rather less reliably.

Many authors, including ourselves, have demonstrated antiarrhythmic protection in rats [7–10,12,13,18], but this is the only species in which consistent protection has been reported and in which the antiarrhythmic properties of ischemic preconditioning are not controversial. Vulnerability to arrhythmias varies widely with species, however, and repeated demonstrations of profound antiarrhythmic protection in dogs by Vegh et al. [10,15,24] have not been confirmed by others [1] and an increase in arrhythmia severity has also been reported [14]. This discrepancy may be a consequence of differences between the studies in the anesthetic agents employed. Vegh et al. [10,15,24] used chloralose and urethane, whereas pentobarbital has been employed for most studies that have failed to show antiarrhythmic protection. Interestingly, Li et al. [25] have also reported a mild reduction in arrhythmia severity following preconditioning in dogs and they also employed a urethane-based anesthetic regimen.

To date there has been only one report of antiarrhythmic activity in pigs [26] and none of antiarrhythmic protection in rabbits. This raises the possibility that preconditioning is not universally protective against arrhythmias but that protection is critically dependent on species. We believe, however, that the inconsistent protection reported is likely to be a consequence of the experimental design employed in many of the studies that failed to demonstrate reductions in arrhythmia severity. Such data are invariably derived from studies designed to study myocardial necrosis or contractile function as their primary end point.

ARRHYTHMOGENESIS AS A SECONDARY END POINT

If preconditioning is to be shown to be effective in preventing arrhythmias, it is important that the design of the experimental protocol should follow certain principles. In this regard, we would suggest that the protocol should:

1. Employ relatively short durations of preconditioning ischemia to limit preconditioning-induced arrhythmias. The precipitation of arrhythmias by the preconditioning protocol is a much less important consideration where

myocardial necrosis is the primary end point, as even life-threatening arrhythmias are generally amenable to direct current cardioversion.

2. Use a large occluded zone to ensure a high incidence of arrhythmias in control hearts during the study period. In our studies with rat hearts this has involved proximal left coronary ligation and the occluded zone has represented over 40% of the ventricular mass. In general, studies of infarct size involve longer experimental durations and thus have employed much smaller occluded zone sizes to limit the number of deaths occurring due to hypotension and cardiac failure.

3. Include a sufficient sample size to allow the identification of a protective effect. In comparison with studies of infarction, larger sample sizes are required to allow the demonstration of a reduction in the incidence of arrhythmias due to differences in the statistical techniques employed. In our arrhythmia studies we generally employ a sample size of 12 per group, whereas it is unusual for the group size to exceed eight in studies of infarct size. For species such as the rabbit in which, even with a large occluded zone, relatively few malignant arrhythmias develop during prolonged coronary occlusion or on reperfusion, much larger group sizes may be required to demonstrate statistically a significant benefit.

4. Use ischemic durations appropriate for the arrhythmia under study. Due to the temporal relationships of ischemia- and reperfusion-induced arrhythmias described above, it is not possible to study both optimally using the same ischemic duration. The analysis of arrhythmia data from infarct size studies has also commonly involved the pooling of data from arrhythmias induced by both ischemia and reperfusion. As the mechanisms involved in ischemia- and reperfusion-induced arrhythmias are widely different, such an approach is of dubious scientific merit.

5. Comply with the Lambeth Conventions [27].

Thus, where arrhythmias are reported as a secondary end point from studies primarily designed to assess infarct size, there is a high probability of underestimating the beneficial antiarrhythmic effects of preconditioning. For this reason we would strongly argue that arrhythmias should be assessed in separate experiments using study protocols specifically designed for that purpose. In addition, ischemia- and reperfusion-induced arrhythmias should, ideally, be studied using distinct experimental protocols. Unfortunately, considerations of cost frequently preclude the strict application of these principles, especially in large animal studies performed in vivo.

WHAT IS THE MECHANISM OF ANTIARRHYTHMIC PROTECTION?

In view of the many similarities between antiarrhythmic and antinecrotic protection by preconditioning, it would be most surprising if the fundamental processes involved were substantially different. Antiarrhythmic protection, however, ultimately must be the manifestation of a preservation of ionic homeostasis, whereas the essential requirements for protection against necrosis may be different. Indeed, from many of the studies outlined above, it is clear that it is possible to protect against necrosis without the prevention of arrhythmias and vice versa. Thus, the detailed mechanisms underlying these separate protective effects may differ.

Cardiac electrophysiology

The effect of sequential coronary occlusions on cardiac electrophysiology has been incompletely explored. Although Gulker et al. [5] have shown that later occlusions are associated with a higher threshold for the precipitation of VF, Fleet et al. [28] have demonstrated a progressive increase in activation delay with sequential coronary occlusions that could actually predispose to the development of reentrant circuits. Conversely, the later occlusions in the study by Fleet et al. [28] were associated with activation block, which could equally interrupt such a circuit. Vegh et al. [16] have shown that antiarrhythmic protection following preconditioning by the induction of transient ischemia by rapid pacing is associated with a reduction in the severity of conduction abnormalities within the ischemic zone. This could limit the dispersion of refractoriness within the ischemic territory and reduce the probability of reentrant circuits developing.

Endogenous protective substances

The few studies that have been performed specifically to identify the molecular mechanisms underlying the antiarrhythmic protection achieved with preconditioning have yielded rather surprising results. Despite a wealth of evidence to suggest an important, and possibly pivotal, role for adenosine in mediating protection against myocardial necrosis in several species [29], there is none to support a role in protection against arrhythmias. This may be due to the majority of studies having been performed in the rat, a species in which adenosine does not appear to be involved in the mechanism of infarct size reduction [22]. Conversely, Vegh et al. [15] showed that antiarrhythmic protection in dogs can be attenuated by the administration of the cyclooxygenase inhibitor meclofenamate. They therefore raised the possibility that preconditioning could be attributed to the production by ischemic myocardium of a prostaglandin analogue. Prostacyclin, which is capable of reducing the severity of ischemia-induced arrhythmias [30], would be a possible candidate for such a role. However, Li et al. [31] found that aspirin failed to prevent protection against both necrosis and ischemia-induced arrhythmias in rats, and Liu et al. [32] have shown that neither meclofenamate nor aspirin prevent protection against infarction in rabbits. The disparity between these results might be explained by differences in species, differences in the protocols employed or the pharmacological agents used, or the possibility of a direct proarrhythmic effect of meclofenamate.

Ionic homeostasis

Potassium

Regional ischemia leads to a variety of proarrhythmic alterations in ionic homeostasis, including the loss of intracellular potassium to the extracellular compartment. The arrhythmogenic potential of regional hyperkalemia is well recognized, but potassium accumulation is not sufficient in itself to precondition against arrhythmias, as repeated episodes of hyperkalemic perfusion elicit repeated arrhythmic episodes [33]. Direct measurement of extracellular potassium with ion-sensitive microelectrodes indicates that, with repeated coronary artery occlusions, the later occlusions lead to a less rapid but ultimately more profound elevation of myocardial extracellular potassium [28]. It is possible that this could have a local cardioplegia-like effect and protect against necrosis. Indeed, Gross and Auchampach have shown that inhibition of the ATP-sensitive potassium channel can prevent protection against myocardial necrosis in dogs [34]. It is difficult to see, however, how enhancement of extracellular potassium accumulation could afford protection against ischemia-induced arrhythmias. In fact ATP-sensitive potassium channel agonists have, in general, been found to be proarrhythmic during ischemia [35]. Activation of ATP-sensitive potassium channels does not appear to be a universal mechanism underlying preconditioning, as pretreatment with glibenclamide does not appear to abolish protection against infarction in rabbits [36] or rats [22].

Calcium

Cellular calcium loading, as a consequence of ischemia and/or reperfusion, may contribute significantly to arrhythmogenesis by a number of proarrhythmic mechanisms, including action potential shortening, the induction of a depolarizing inward current, and impaired intracellular conduction [37,38]. Nuclear magnetic resonance studies have indicated that ischemia-induced calcium loading is profoundly reduced by preconditioning [39]. Hypoxic perfusion appears to be as effective as ischemia in inducing preconditioning [40,41] and also limits the uptake of radiolabelled calcium [42]. It is possible therefore, that the antiarrhythmic actions of preconditioning might be a consequence of its modulation of cellular calcium loading, but if so it remains far from clear how this modulation occurs.

Protons

Proton washout can lead to an exacerbation of ischemia-induced sodium loading upon reperfusion (by sodium–proton exchange) and consequent calcium loading due to sodium–calcium exchange [42,43]. Proton washout may, therefore, be important in the initiation of reperfusion-induced arrhythmias. Support for this concept has been provided by Avkiran and Ibuki [44], who have recently shown that acidic reperfusion can prevent reperfusion-induced arrhythmias by attenuating the sudden development of a proton gradient across the sarcolemmal membrane. Direct measurement of extracellular pH, and measurement of intracellular pH by NMR spectroscopy, have shown reductions in both with serial ischemic episodes [28,45]. This could lead to an amelioration of reperfusion-induced arrhythmias by reducing the transsarcolemmal proton gradient produced by extracellular proton washout on reperfusion.

Oxidant stress

The cellular mechanisms underlying reperfusion-induced arrhythmias appear to be substantially different from those responsible for the induction of ischemia-induced arrhythmias. A number of authors have emphasized the importance of oxidant stress in the precipitation of reperfusion-induced arrhythmias [46,47], but there have been conflicting reports on the effect of preconditioning on tissue antioxidant defenses [48,49], and no direct measurements of the effect of preconditioning on free radical production have been made. Prevention of preconditioning-mediated antiarrhythmic protection by free-radical scavengers has been demonstrated by Osada et al. [12], but, as described previously, the design of this study was not ideal. Free radical scavengers do not appear to prevent preconditioning from protecting against myocardial necrosis [50].

Autonomic dysfunction

It is well established that ischemia and reperfusion can lead to a substantial depletion of noradrenaline stores from cardiac sympathetic nerve terminals. Shiki and Hearse [7] suggested that the depletion of endogenous catecholamines, as a consequence of preconditioning, might protect the heart during subsequent episodes of ischemia and reperfusion. Indeed, pharmacological depletion of endogenous catecholamines can induce marked protection against reperfusion-induced arrhythmias [51]. However, evidence from a number of sources suggests that catecholamine depletion is not the mechanism by which preconditioning affords antiarrhythmic protection. We have measured myocardial catecholamine levels before and after preconditioning and following a prolonged ischemic episode. Although preconditioning provided marked protection against ischemia-induced arrhythmias, it did not lead to significant depletion of myocardial catecholamines. In addition, the rate of depletion during prolonged ischemia was unaffected (unpublished data). Indirect evidence that brief cycles of ischemia and reperfusion are not associated with significant catecholamine depletion is provided by Janes [52], who showed that the effect of stellate ganglion stimulation is preserved after 12 cycles of 5 minutes of ischemia and reperfusion.

On the contrary, Miyazaki and Zipes [53] have shown that in a canine model of preconditioning both sympathetic and parasympathetic reflexes are actually *preserved* during ischemia. It is possible that this preservation of autonomic function might contribute to protection against ischemia-induced arrhythmias by reducing heterogeneity between innervated and denervated regions. Although it would be possible for such a mechanism to be operative in vivo, it could not account for the protection reported in isolated heart preparations. Thus it is unlikely that the preservation of autonomic reflexes or the depletion of endogenous catecholamines play significant roles in the antiarrhythmic action of ischemic preconditioning.

Signal transduction

Although there is currently little evidence to suggest that adenosine plays a direct role in mediating the antiarrhythmic actions of preconditioning, many of the actions of adenosine A_1 receptors are mediated via inhibitory G_i proteins [54], which are also central to the signal transduction of a number of other membrane receptors, including the muscarinic M_2 receptor [55]. Transient stimulation of the M_2 receptor has been reported to mimic preconditioning [56]. This raises the possibility that G_i proteins might mediate a common mechanism for the diverse protective actions of preconditioning.

Pertussis toxin, which blocks the coupling of G_i proteins to membrane receptors, can prevent preconditioning from protecting against infarction in rabbits [57]. Piacientini et al. [58] have recently reported that pertussis toxin pretreatment can prevent antiarrhythmic protection by preconditioning in isolated crystalloid-perfused rat hearts. This result, however, conflicts directly with those of a similar study of our own [59] performed in isolated rat hearts perfused with blood. We found no evidence that pertussis-toxin pretreatment could prevent preconditioning from protecting against ischemia -induced arrhythmias in our model. The explanation for these contradictory results is not clear, but presumably must relate to the nature of the different perfusates employed. Our results accord with those of Liu et al. [60] who have recently shown that protection against myocardial necrosis in rats in vivo is not prevented by pertussis toxin pretreatment. Thus it appears that, both in vivo and in isolated hearts perfused with blood, functional G_i proteins are not involved in the protective effects of preconditioning in rats.

Vegh et al. [24] have reported that N^G-nitro-L-arginine methyl esther hydrochloride (L-NAME), an inhibitor of nitric oxide synthesis, can partially attenuate the protective actions of preconditioning on ischemia-induced arrhythmias and ischemia-induced inhomogeneity of conduction. As nitric oxide acts by stimulating soluble guanylyl cyclase, they have speculated that these protective effects may be mediated by an elevation of cyclic GMP. Analogues of cyclic GMP have been shown to have potent antiarrhythmic actions in dogs [61], and recent data suggest that methylene blue, which inhibits guanylyl cyclase, can reverse the antiarrhythmic action of preconditioning in dogs [62]. It is possible, however, that methylene blue might have a direct proarrhythmic effect rather than acting to prevent preconditioning per se. The effector mechanisms that might mediate the antiarrhythmic actions of an elevated cyclic GMP level are currently not clear, although possibilities include modulation of cytosolic calcium levels and sarcoplasmic potassium channels.

Can ischemia be antiarrhythmic?

It has been suggested that the precipitation of arrhythmias by reperfusion is not a consequence of a direct arrhythmic property of reperfusion per se but due instead to the loss of an antiarrhythmic property of ischemia [63]. Although ischemia clearly induces arrhythmias it provides a complex insult to the myocardium, and it is possible that some component(s) of ischemia may be antiarrhythmic. Support for this concept is provided by the observation that ischemia is capable of terminating pharmacologically induced arrhythmias [64]. The nature of this putative antiarrhythmic component of ischemia remains entirely speculative, and it has yet to be demonstrated that any specific component of an ischemic challenge can persist through a period of reperfusion and be sufficiently long-lived to underlie the antiarrhythmic action of preconditioning.

CLINICAL RELEVANCE OF ANTIARRHYTHMIC PROTECTION

The possibility that preconditioning might be amenable to clinical exploitation is being explored following the report by Deutch et al. [65] that, at least in the context of balloon angioplasty, preconditioning is capable of reducing the apparent severity of ischemia in humans during the early phase of coronary artery occlusion. Mortality in the very early stages of acute myocardial infarction is believed to be more commonly due to the precipitation of malignant arrhythmias than to pump failure. Patients developing such malignant arrhythmias in the early phase of infarction will die suddenly unless medical intervention is immediately available on site. Indeed, death prior to arrival at hospital remains the major obstacle to reducing further the current mortality rate of acute infarction. In addition, sudden cardiac death occurring in patients with coronary artery disease or coronary artery spasm in the absence of infarction is also believed to be due to malignant arrhythmias. Conventional pharmacological antiarrhythmic therapy is generally unsatisfactory for the treatment of ischemia- and reperfusion-induced malignant arrhythmias and has yet to be demonstrated to have any beneficial effect on mortality in patients with ischemic heart disease. As a result, nonpharmacological modalities for patients with life-threatening arrhythmias are currently being extensively explored, such as implantable defibrillators, catheter ablation, and antiarrhythmic surgery.

When the molecular mechanisms underlying preconditioning have been determined, it may then be possible to offer these patients powerful and effective pharmacological protection against arrhythmias occurring in the setting of acute ischemia and reperfusion. In addition, if preconditioning can be shown to be effective in other models of arrhythmogenesis, it may be possible to offer improved pharmacological therapy to patients with arrhythmias of diverse etiologies.

CONCLUDING COMMENTS

Over and above its antiischemic actions, preconditioning has a powerful antiarrhythmic effect. If this antiarrhythmic property is to be adequately analyzed, it is essential that studies should be designed to look specifically at its mechanisms using appropriate models and experimental protocols. Design of such protocols is more complicated than for infarct size studies. Not only is it desirable that the preconditioning protocol should precipitate as few arrhythmias as possible, but it is also essential that the preconditioning protocol should not lead to spurious protection as a consequence of cumulative irreversible ischemic damage.

There are a number of features that indicate that protection against arrhythmias might be qualitatively different from that against necrosis. These include its dose dependency, the lack of effect of preconditioning on the temporal pattern of arrhythmogenesis, and the possibility of differences in the molecular mechanisms involved. In addition, antiarrhythmic protection provides the only firm evidence to date that preconditioning can protect against reversible as well as irreversible myocardial injury. As it remains far from clear that the diverse protective effects of preconditioning are mediated by common mechanisms, it is essential when reporting results that both the preconditioning stimulus and the primary end point under study should be specified.

REFERENCES

1. Murry CE, Jennings RB, Reimer KA. 1986. Preconditioning with ischemia: A delay of lethal cell injury in ischemic myocardium. Circulation 74:1124–1136.
2. Lawson CS, Downey JM. 1993. Preconditioning: State of the art myocardial protection. Cardiovasc Res:542–550.
3. Neely JR, Grotyohan LV. 1984. Role of glycolytic products in damage to the ischemic myocardium: Dissociation of adenosine triphosphate levels and recovery of reperfused ischemic hearts. Circ Res 55:816–824.
4. Harris AS. 1950. Delayed development of ventricular ectopic rhythms following experimental coronary occlusion. Circulation 1:1318–1327.
5. Gulker J, Kramer B, Stephan K, Meeseman W. 1977. Changes in ventricular fibrillation threshold during repeated short-term coronary occlusion and release. Basic Res Cardiol 72:547–562.
6. Barber MJ. 1983. Effect of time interval between repeated brief coronary artery occlusions on arrhythmia, electrical activity and myocardial blood flow. J Am Coll Cardiol 2:699–705.
7. Shiki K, Hearse DJ. 1987. Preconditioning of ischemic myocardium: Reperfusion-induced arrhythmias. Am J Physiol 253:H1470–H1476.
8. Li YW, Whittaker P, Kloner RA. 1992. The transient nature of the effect of ischemic preconditioning on myocardial infarct size and ventricular arrhythmia. Am Heart J 123: 346–353.
9. Hagar JM, Hale SL, Kloner RA. 1991. Effects of preconditioning ischemia on reperfusion arrhythmias after coronary artery occlusion and reperfusion in the rat. Circ Res 68:61–68.

10. Vegh A, Komoro S, Szekeres L, Parratt JR. 1992. Antiarrhythmic effects of preconditioning in anaesthetised dogs and rats. Cardiovasc Res 26:487–495.
11. Manning AS, Hearse DJ. 1984. Reperfusion-induced arrhythmias: Mechanisms and prevention. J Mol Cell Cardiol 16:497–518.
12. Osada M, Sato T, Tamura K. 1991. Protective effect of preconditioning on reperfusion induced ventricular arrhythmias of isolated rat hearts. Cardiovasc Res 25:441–444.
13. Lawson CS, Coltart DJ, Hearse DJ. 1992. Ischaemic preconditioning and reperfusion-induced arrhythmias: Reduction in vulnerability or delay in onset? Studies in the isolated blood-perfused rat heart. Eur Heart J 13(Suppl):401 (abstr).
14. Reimer KA, Murry CE, Jennings RB. 1990. Cardiac adaptation to ischemia. Ischemic preconditioning increases myocardial tolerance to subsequent ischemic episodes. Circulation 82:2266–2268.
15. Vegh A, Szekeres L, Parratt JR. 1990. Protective effects of preconditioning of the ischaemic myocardium involve cyclo-oxygenase products. Cardiovasc Res 24:1020–1023.
16. Vegh A, Szekeres L, Parratt JR. 1991. Transient ischaemia induced by rapid pacing results in myocardial preconditioning. Cardiovasc Res 25:1051–1053.
17. Marber MS, Walker DM, Yellon DM, Walker M. 1992. Rapid atrial pacing fails to precondition the rabbit heart. J Mol Cell Cardiol 24(Suppl I):92 (abstr).
18. Lawson CS, Hearse DJ. 1992. Ischaemic preconditioning reduces rather than delays early ischaemia-induced arrhythmias in the isolated blood-perfused rat heart. J Mol Cell Cardiol 24(Suppl V):S88 (abstr).
19. Lawson CS, Coltart DJ, Hearse DJ. 1992. Ischaemic preconditioning and reperfusion-induced arrhythmias: Reduction in vulnerability or delay in onset? Studies in the isolated blood-perfused rat heart. Eur Heart J 13(Suppl):401 (abstr).
20. Miura T, Ogawa T, Iwamoto T. 1990. Infarct size limiting effect of preconditioning: Its duration and "dose-response" relationship. Circulation 83(Suppl III):271 (abstr).
21. Van Winkle DM, Thornton J, Downey JM. 1991. Cardioprotection from ischemic preconditioning is lost following prolonged reperfusion in the rabbit. Coron Artery Dis 2: 613–619.
22. Liu Y, Downey JM. 1992 Ischaemic preconditioning protects against infarction in rat heart. Am J Physiol 263:H1107–H1112.
23. Walker DM, Yellon DM. 1992. Ischaemic preconditioning: From mechanism to exploitation. Cardiovasc Res 26:734–739.
24. Vegh A, Szekeres L, Parratt JR. 1992. Preconditioning of the ischaemic myocardium: Involvement of the L-arginine nitric oxide pathway. Br J Pharmacol 107:648–625.
25. Li GC, Vasquez JA, Gallagher KP, Lucchesi BR. 1990. Myocardial protection with preconditioning. Circulation 82:609–619.
26. Wainwright CL, Parratt JR. 1990. Electrocardiographic and haemodynamic effects of myocardial preconditioning in pigs. J Mol Cell Cardiol 22(Suppl III):S77 (abstr).
27. Walker MJA, Curtis MJ, Hearse DJ. 1988. The Lambeth Conventions: Guidelines for the study of arrhythmias in ischaemia, infarction and reperfusion. Cardiovasc Res 22: 447–455.
28. Fleet WF, Johnson TA, Graebner CA, Gettes LS. 1985. Effect of serial brief ischemic episodes on extracellular K, pH and activation in the pig. Circulation 2:922–932.
29. Mullane K. 1992. Myocardial preconditioning. Part of the adenosine revival. Circulation 85:845–847.
30. Coker SJ, Parratt JR. 1983. Prostacyclin-antiarrhythmic or arrhythmogenic? Comparison of the effects of intravenous and intracoronary prostacyclin and ZX 36374 during coronary artery occlusion and reperfusion in the anaesthetised greyhound. J Cardiovasc Pharmacol 5:557–567.
31. Li Y, Kloner RA. 1992. Cardioprotective effects of ischaemic preconditioning are not mediated by prostanoids. Cardiovasc Res 26:226–231.
32. Liu GS, Stanley AHS, Downey JM. 1992. Cyclooxygenase products are not involved in the protection against myocardial infarction afforded by preconditioning in rabbit. Am J Cardiovasc Pathol 4:56–63.
33. Curtis MJ. 1991. The rabbit dual coronary perfusion model: A new method for assessing the pathological relevance of individual products of the ischaemic milieu: Role of potassium in arrhythmogenesis. Cardiovasc Res 25:1010–1022.

34. Gross GJ, Auchampach JA. 1992. Blockade of ATP-sensitive potassium channel prevents myocardial preconditioning in dogs. Circ Res 70:223–233.
35. Coetzee WA. 1992. ATP-sensitive potassium channels and myocardial ischemia: Why do they open? Cardiovasc Drugs Ther 6:201–208.
36. Thornton J, Downey JM. 1993. Blockade of ATP-sensitive potassium channels increases infarct size but does not prevent preconditioning in rabbit hearts. Circ Res 72:44–49.
37. Clusin WT, Buchbinder M, Bristow MR, Harrison DC. 1984. Evidence for a role of calcium in the genesis of early ischemic cardiac arrhythmias. In Calcium Antagonists and Cardiovascular Disease, L Opie, ed. Raven Press, New York, pp. 293–302.
38. Opie LH, Coetzee WA. 1988. Role of calcium ions in reperfusion arrhythmias: Relevance to pharmacological intervention. Cardiovasc Drugs Ther 2:623–636.
39. Steenbergen C, Perlman ME, London RE, Murphy E. 1993. Mechanism of preconditioning: Ionic alterations. Circ Res 72:112–125.
40. Zhai X, Lawson CS, Hearse DJ. 1992. Are ischemia and hypoxia equivalent preconditioning stimuli in the isolated rat heart? Circulation 86(Suppl I):31 (abstr).
41. Shizukida Y, Mallet RT, Lee S-C, Downey HF. 1992. Hypoxic preconditioning of ischaemic canine myocardium. Cardiovas Res 26:534–542.
42. Tani M, Neely JR. 1989. Role of intracellular Na^+ in Ca^{2+} overload and depressed recovery of ventricular function of reperfused ischemic rat hearts. Circ Res 65:1045–1056.
43. Lazdunski M, Frelin C, Vigne P. 1985. The sodium/hydrogen exchange system is cardiac cells: Its biological and pharmacological properties and its role in regulating internal concentrations of sodium and internal pH. J Mol Cell Cardiol 17:1029–1042.
44. Avkiran M, Ibuki C. 1992. Reperfusion-induced arrhythmias: A role for washout of extracellular protons? Circ Res 71:1429–1440.
45. Kida M, Fujiwara H, Ishida M, Kawai C, Ohura M, Miura I, Yabuuchi Y. 1991. Ischemic preconditioning preserves creatine phosphate and intracellular pH. Circulation 84:2495–2503.
46. Bernier M, Hearse DJ, Manning AS. 1986. Reperfusion induced arrhythmias and oxygen-derived free radicals. Studies with anti-free radical interventions and a free radical generating system in the isolated perfused rat heart. Circ Res 58:331–340.
47. Woodward B, Zakaria MVM. 1985. Effect of some free radical scavangers on reperfusion-induced arrhythmias in the isolated rat heart. J Mol Cell Cardiol 17:L485–493.
48. Hoshida S, Kuzuya T, Fuji H, Oe H, Kimura Y, Sasaki T, Kitabatake A, Tada M. 1991. Ischemic preconditioning affects free radical generating and scavenging systems in canine myocardial infarction. Circulation 84(Suppl II):192 (abstr).
49. Turrens JF, Thornton J, Barnard ML, Snyder S, Liu G, Downey JM. 1992. Protection from reperfusion injury by preconditioning hearts does not involve increased antioxidant defenses. Am J Physiol 262:H585–589.
50. Iwamoto T, Miura T, Adechi T, Noto T, Ogawa T, Tsuchida A, Iimura O. 1991. Myocardial infarct size-limiting effect of ischemic preconditioning was not attenuated by oxygen free-radical scavengers in the rabbit. Circulation 83:1015–1022.
51. Manning AS, Crome R, Lewis MJ, J SM, Hearse DJ. 1988. Myocardial ischaemia and life threatening arrhythmias: Protective effects of chronic prenylamine administration. In Prenylamine: A Novel Approach to Myocardial Protection, AS Manning, GL Szendey, eds. Raven Press, New York, pp. 63–73.
52. Janes RD, Johnstone DE, Klassen GA, Armour JA. 1985. The function of cardiac sympathetic efferent nerves within a zone of repeated ischemia. Circulation 72(Suppl III):63 (abstr).
53. Miyazaki T, Zipes DP. 1989. Protection against autonomic denervation following acute myocardial infarction by preconditioning ischemia. Circ Res 64:437–448.
54. Stiles GL. 1991. Adenosine receptors: Physiologic regulation and biochemical mechanisms. NIPS 6:161–165.
55. Birnbaumer L, Abramowitz J, Brown AM. 1990. Receptor-effector coupling by G proteins. Biochim Biophys Acta 1031:163–224.
56. Lasley RD, Van Wylen DGL, Mentzer RM. 1990. Evidence for the role of Gi proteins in attenuating myocardial ischemic damage. Circulation 82(Suppl III):759 (abstr).
57. Thornton JD, Downey JM. 1993. Pretreatment with pertussis toxin blocks the protective effects of preconditioning: Evidence for a Gi-protein mechanism. J Mol Cell Cardiol 25:311–320.

58. Piacientini L, Wainwright C, Parratt JR. 1992. Prevention of the antiarrhythmic effects of ischaemic preconditioning by pertussis toxin pretreatment. J Mol Cell Cardiol 24(Suppl V):S92 (abstr).
59. Lawson CS, Coltart DJ, Hearse DJ. 1993. The anti-arrhythmic action of ischemic preconditioning in rat hearts does not involve functional Gi proteins. Cardiovasc Res 27:681–687.
60. Liu Y, Downey JM. 1993. Preconditioning against infarction in the rat heart does not involve a pertussis toxin-sensitive G protein. Cardiovasc Res 27:608–611.
61. Billman GE. 1990. Effect of carbachol and cyclic GMP on susceptibility to ventricular fibrillation. FASEB J 4:1668–1673.
62. Vegh A, Papp JG, Szekeres L, Parratt JR. The local intracoronary administration of methylene blue prevents the pronounced antiarrhythmic effect of ischaemic preconditioning. Br J Pharmacol, in press.
63. Nakata T, Hearse DJ, Curtis MJ. 1990. Are reperfusion-induced arrhythmias caused by disinhibition of an arrhythmogenic component of ischemia? J Mol Cell Cardiol 22:843–858.
64. Podzuweit T, Binz K-H. 1989. The anti-arhythmic effects of myocardial ischaemia. Relation to reperfusion arrhythmias. Cardiovasc Res 23:81–90.
65. Deutsch E, Berger M, Kussmaul WG, Hirshfeld JWJ, Herrmann HC, Laskey MD. 1990. Adaptation to ischemia during percutaneous transluminal coronary angioplasty. Clinical, hemodynamic and metabolic features. Circulation 82:2044–2051.

3. PRECONDITIONING AND MYOCARDIAL CONTRACTILE FUNCTION

MICHEL OVIZE, ROBERT A. KLONER, and KARIN PRZYKLENK

INTRODUCTION

Hearts exposed to a reversible ischemic insult become more resistant to a subsequent more prolonged episode of coronary artery occlusion, i.e., they develop significantly smaller infarcts. This endogenous protection has been termed *preconditioning* [1]. While this reduction in infarct size with preconditioning has been confirmed in numerous experimental models, the relationship between preconditioning and contractile function remains less well defined. Two specific aspects of this issue have generated interest and controversy. First, as brief episodes of ischemia/reperfusion cause transient hypokinesis or stunning, does stunning represent the mechanism for reduction in infarct size by preconditioning? Secondly, is this reduction in infarct size accompanied by improved contractile performance of the salvaged myocardium following relief of sustained ischemia? In the present chapter we will discuss the relationship between preconditioning and contractile function, with special attention to the possible confounding role of irreversible cellular injury and to apparent differences among experimental preparations.

IS PRECONDITIONING A CONSEQUENCE OF STUNNING?

Myocardium that has undergone brief episodes of ischemia/reperfusion is "preconditioned". This tissue also exhibits wall motion abnormalities refered to as *stunning*. One approach to evaluate a possible cause-and-effect relationship between preconditioning and stunning is to determine whether the two phenomena can be dissociated from one another, i.e., is it possible to alter one phenomenon without modifying the other one? Various attempts have been made that, taken together, strongly suggest that preconditioning is not a consequence of myocardial stunning.

Dissociation of the time course of the two phenomena

Murry et al. have demonstrated that preconditioning is associated with a reduction of adenosine triphoshate (ATP) utilization during the first 15 minutes of sustained ischemia in the dog [2]. They hypothesized that stunning resulting from the initial brief ischemic episode might limit myocardial energy demand during the subsequent prolonged ischemia, and thereby preserve cellular viability [3]. Moreover, Shröder et al. have demonstrated that contractile activity decreases slightly but significantly faster (and might thereby result in further sparing of ATP) during a second episode of reversible ischemia than during the first one [4]. If this line of reasoning were correct, then protection afforded by preconditioning would last as long as stunning persists.

To test this concept, Murry and colleagues designed an experimental protocol aimed at comparing the time courses of stunning and preconditioning [3]. Briefly, three groups of dogs underwent 40 minutes of prolonged coronary artery occlusion followed by 4 days of reperfusion. Control dogs received no intervention, while the two preconditioned groups underwent 15

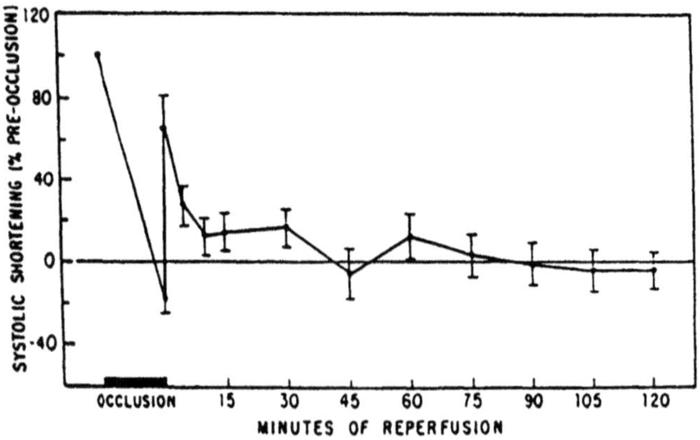

Figure 1. Regional contractile function during the preconditioning phase. Data were obtained from dogs with subendocardial collateral blood flow ≤0.15 ml/min/g. Segment shortening (expressed as percentage of baseline values) is presented during the 15-minute preconditioning ischemia and the following 2 hours of reperfusion preceding the prolonged coronary artery occlusion. The ischemic/reperfused region exhibited severe stunning (akinesia) for the 2 hours prior to the sustained ischemic insult. Reprinted from Murry et al. [3], with permission of the American Physiological Society.

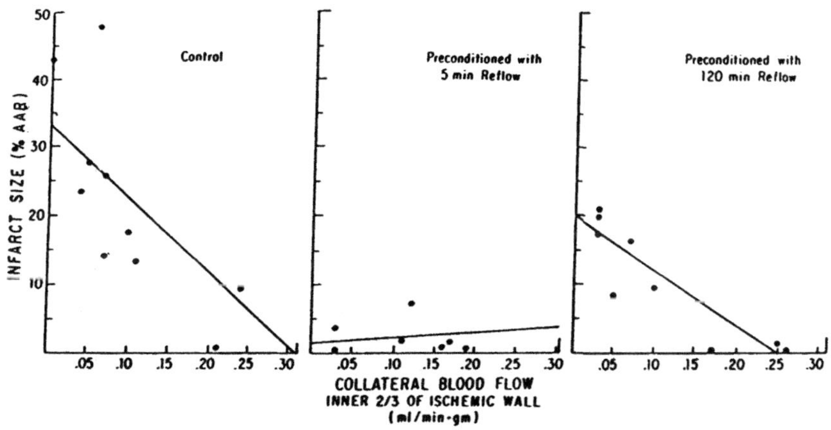

Figure 2. Infarct size as a function of collateral flow. In control hearts subjected to 40 minutes of sustained coronary artery occlusion, there was an inverse relationship between collateral blood flow and infarct size; i.e., hearts with low collateral flow had large infarcts and vice versa. In the preconditioned group with 5 minutes of intervening reperfusion, infarcts were smaller than control at any level of collateral flow ($p < 0.01$ by analysis of covariance). In the preconditioned group with 120 minutes of intervening reflow, the regression line was intermediate between that of the control and 5-minute reperfusion groups ($p < 0.05$ vs. control; $p < 0.01$ vs. 5-minute reperfusion group). This indicates that extending the duration of reperfusion between preconditioning and sustained occlusion to 2 hours significantly attenuated preconditioning's protective effect. AAR = area at risk of infarction. Reprinted from Murry et al. [3], with permission of the American Physiological Society.

minutes of ischemia followed either by 5 minutes or 2 hours of intervening reperfusion before the prolonged ischemic insult. As expected, 15 minutes of brief preconditioning ischemia resulted in prolonged postischemic stunning, with no improvement in segment shortening during the first 2 hours of reflow (Figure 1). However, the reduction in infarct size achieved with preconditioning was greater in dogs reperfused for only 5 minutes prior to the sustained ischemia than in dogs in which the intervening period of reperfusion was maintained for 2 hours (Figure 2). This 2-hour delay did not, however, fully abolish the protective effect of the brief ischemia. In the "2-hour delay" preconditioned group, mean infarct size (expressed as percentage of the risk region) averaged 12%, significantly larger than the value of 2% in the "5-minute delay" preconditioned group ($p < 0.05$), but still significantly smaller than the value of 27% in the control group ($p < 0.01$).

Thus, Murry et al. demonstrated that, despite persistent stunning due to the preceding brief ischemia, the protective effect of preconditioning is attenuated, but not fully abolished, when the intervening reperfusion period between brief ischemia and the sustained ischemia is prolonged to 2 hours. This study, therefore, suggests that the time course of stunning differs from that of preconditioning.

Similar cardioprotection for different degrees of stunning

Miura et al. chose to address the relationship between stunning and preconditioning from a different angle. These authors sought to determine whether different degrees of stunning (achieved by manipulating the episodes of brief preconditioning ischemia) would afford similar reduction in infarct size [5].

Three preconditioning regimens, aimed at varying contractile dysfunction in the ischemic/reperfused myocardium, were compared. Specifically, rabbits received either two episodes of 2 minutes of ischemia separated by 5 minutes of reperfusion (2′ PC group), one episode of 5 minutes of ischemia followed by 5 minutes of reperfusion (5′ PC_1 group), two episodes of 5 minutes of ischemia separated by 5 minutes of reperfusion (5′ PC_2 group), or no intervention (control group). All animals then underwent 30 minutes of sustained coronary artery occlusion followed by 72 hours of reperfusion. As expected, wall thickening (WT) in the preconditioned myocardium was significantly lower in rabbits that underwent one or two episodes of 5-minute ischemia/reperfusion (WT averaged 32–35% of baseline values) when compared with those that received two episodes of 2 minutes of ischemia (WT averaged 75% of baseline values). Yet, reduction in infarct size was similar in all three groups, averaging half the area of necrosis observed in the control group. Thus, different degrees of stunning induced by different preconditioning regimens did not result in different degrees of infarct size reduction.

Miura et al. concluded that preconditioning was not a consequence of stunning. However, it should be noted that wall thickening was slightly depressed (to 75% of baseline values) in rabbits preconditioned by two episodes of 2 minutes of ischemia: It remains possible that this mild stunning may have been sufficient to trigger a tolerance to further sustained ischemia. In addition, both the severity of postischemic contractile dysfunction and the extent of necrosis in this rabbit model are dependent upon the size of the area at risk [6]. In the study by Miura and colleagues, the area at risk (expressed as percentage of heart weight) averaged 15% in rabbits preconditioned by two episodes of 2 minutes of ischemia vs. 19% in groups preconditioned by one or two episodes of 5 minutes of ischemia. Although not statistically significant, this difference may have attenuated the severity of stunning in the 2′ PC group. This study does, however, provide convincing evidence that different degrees of stunning produced by different preconditioning regimens result in similar infarct size reduction. This suggests that the two phenomena are likely not related with respect to their intensity.

Preconditioning without previous stunning

Li et al. have previously demonstrated that one episode of 5 minutes of preconditioning ischemia was sufficient to induce subsequent infarct size reduction [7]. As part of a recent study, we evaluated whether one episode of 2.5 minutes of coronary artery occlusion followed by 5 minutes of reflow

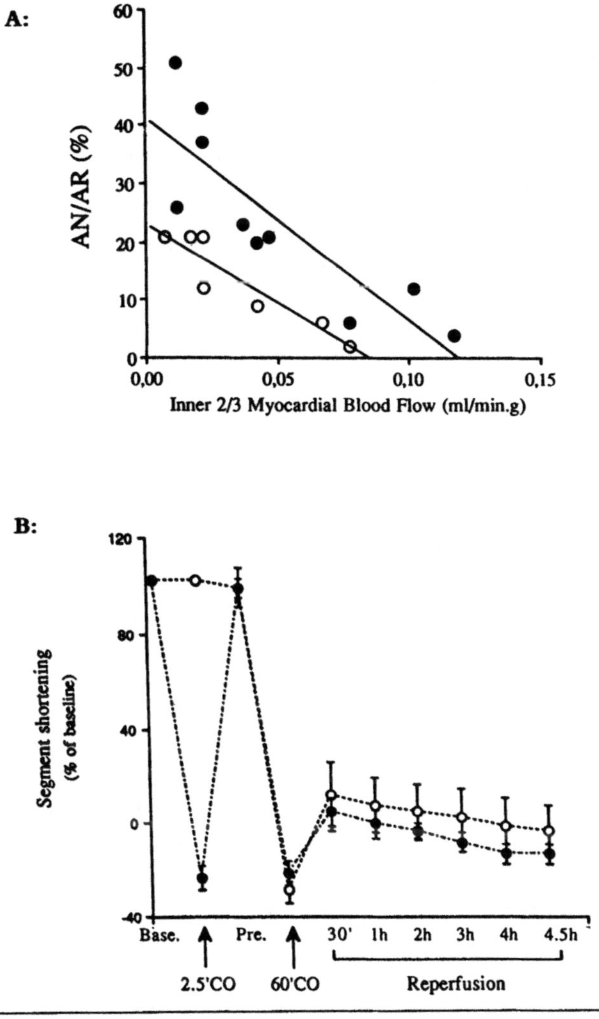

Figure 3. Preconditioning with one *very brief* episode of ischemia. **A:** Infarct size (expressed as a percentage of area at risk) is plotted vs. collateral blood flow during the 1-hour period of prolonged coronary artery occlusion for control (filled circles) and preconditioned (open circles) groups. There was an inverse relationship between collateral blood flow and infarct size in both groups. The regression line for the 2.5-minute preconditioned group was shifted downward with respect to the control line, indicating that for any level of collateral flow, 2.5 minutes of ischemia significantly reduced infarct size ($p < 0.05$ by analysis of covariance). AR = area at risk; AN = area of necrosis. **B:** Segment shortening (expressed as percentage of baseline values) was monitored throughout the experiment in control (filled circles) and 2.5-minute-preconditioned (open circles) groups. Note that just prior to the 60-minute coronary artery occlusion (Pre.) preconditioned hearts did not exhibit stunning. Moreover, the preconditioned and control groups exhibited similar contractile dysfunction during the initial 4.5 hours of reflow following the 60-minute ischemic insult. Base. = baseline; CO = coronary occlusion. Reprinted from Ovize et al. [8] with permission of the American Heart Association.

was sufficient to precondition the canine myocardium [8]. Control and preconditioned groups had similar area at risk and similar collateral blood flow during the prolonged 1 hour ischemia. One episode of 2.5 minutes of ischemia did induce preconditioning: Infarct size averaged 12% of the area at risk in the preconditioned group vs. 25% in the control group ($p < 0.05$, Figure 3A). Interestingly, following 2.5 minutes of ischemia and 5 minutes of reperfusion (i.e., just prior to the prolonged coronary artery occlusion), segment shortening (assessed by sonomicrometry) was maintained at 92% of baseline values in the preconditioned group vs. 97% in the control group (p = NS; Figure 3B). Thus, preconditioning had been induced in the absence of stunning prior to the prolonged ischemic insult.

Another study from our group supports the idea that preconditioning is not a consequence of stunning [9]. Our objective was to determine whether stretch, produced by acute volume overload, might induce preconditioning in the absence of ischemia. Using the canine model, hearts were dilated by rapid infusion of 500 ml saline into the left atrium over 10 minutes, followed by a 10-minute "no intervention" period. As a consequence of this acute volume overload, end-diastolic segment length increased to 115 ± 2% of baseline values in the soon-to-be ischemic area. Hearts that received this treatment developed significantly smaller infarcts as compared with control: Infarct size (expressed as percentage of the area at risk) averaged 15% in the volume-loaded group vs. 32% in the control group ($p < 0.01$). In contrast to the regional hypokinesis exhibited in hearts conventionally preconditioned by ischemia, contractile function did not deteriorate in hearts "preconditioned" by stretch: Immediately prior to the prolonged coronary artery occlusion, segment shortening was 110% of baseline values (p = NS vs. baseline). Thus, infarct size was significantly smaller in hearts preconditioned by stretch, despite the absence of stunning prior to the prolonged ischemic insults. These results, together with our previous study [8], suggest that in the canine heart reduction in infarct size with preconditioning is not dependent upon stunning induced by the preconditioning regimen.

Pharmacological dissociation of stunning and preconditioning

In a preliminary study, Rohmann et al. demonstrated that preconditioning could be induced even when stunning was attenuated by nifedipine (10). Specifically, swine hearts were preconditioned by 10 minutes of ischemia followed by 30 minutes of reperfusion. Nifedipine (5 μg/kg/min), administered during the preconditioning phase, effectively prevented the postischemic dysfunction due to the 10 minutes of brief ischemia, yet infarct size following sustained ischemia was significantly smaller than that observed in the control group.

Other studies indirectly support this concept that stunning and preconditioning may be pharmacologically dissociated. As described earlier, we recently "preconditioned" canine hearts by acute volume overload [9]. We further found that protection induced both by volume overload and by conventional ischemic preconditioning could be blunted by Gd^{3+} (a potent blocker of stretch-activated ion channels). Yet, Gd^{3+} had no significant effect on contractile function. Thus, preconditioning was attenuated by a substance that did not affect contractile function in general, and stunning preceding the prolonged ischemic insult in particular. Similarly, other pharmacologic agents that in some models appear to block preconditioning (adenosine A_1 antagonists, blockers of ATP-sensitive K^+ channels) do not appear to alter contractile function [11,12].

In summary, these studies allow us to conclude that (1) preconditioning and stunning have different time courses, (2) different degrees of stunning are associated with similar infarct size reduction, (3) preconditioning can be induced in the absence of previous stunning, and (4) pharmacological inhibition of one of the two phenomena does not significantly interfere with the other one. Taken together, these observations strongly suggest that preconditioning is not a consequence of stunning.

DOES PRECONDITIONING IMPROVE RECOVERY OF POSTISCHEMIC CONTRACTILE DYSFUNCTION IN IN-SITU PREPARATIONS?

Myocyte necrosis is not the only consequence of sustained ischemia; coronary occlusion/reperfusion also results in ventricular arrhythmias, vascular damage, and myocardial stunning, the incidence of which are determined largely by the severity of the previous ischemic insult. Studies have shown that preconditioning significantly reduces the incidence of ventricular tachycardia and ventricular fibrillation in the rat model [13–15]. One might also ask whether preconditioning favorably influences contractile performance of the viable, previously ischemic tissue. This issue is of considerable importance since contractile dysfunction following acute myocardial infarction is an important determinant of prognosis in humans.

Does preconditioning improve recovery of contractile function after acute myocardial infarction?

We recently sought to determine whether preconditioning could improve the recovery of contractile function (monitored by sonomicrometry) during the 4.5 hours of reperfusion following a 1-hour ischemic insult in the dog [16]. One group of dogs preconditioned by four episodes of (3 minutes of LAD coronary artery occlusion + 5 minutes of reflow) was compared to a control group that received no intervention before the prolonged ischemia. The extent of myocardium at risk, as well as collateral blood flow during the 60-minute coronary occlusion, were similar in the two groups, but, as expected, preconditioned hearts developed significantly smaller infarcts when compared with control (Figure 4A). However, preconditioned and control groups exhibited similar postischemic contractile dysfunction throughout reperfusion (Figure 4B); i.e., at 4.5 hours after relief of ischemia, segment shortening

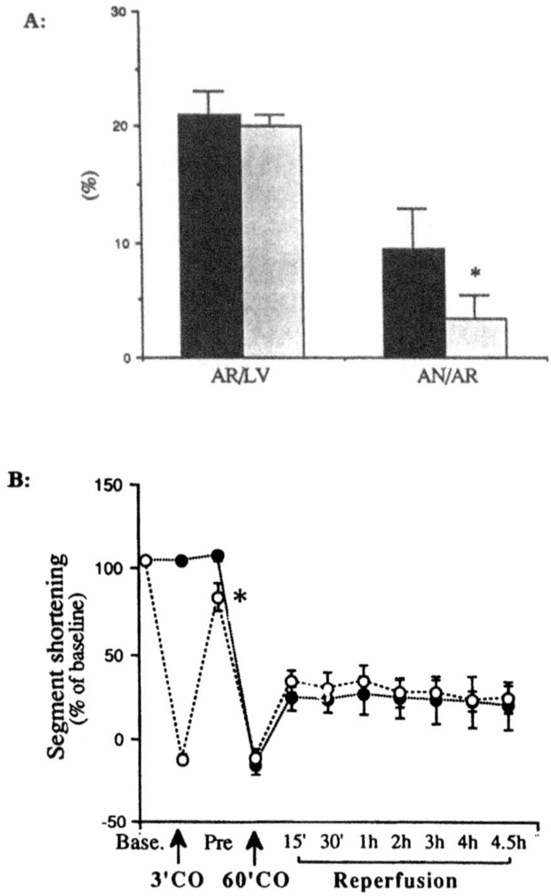

Figure 4. **A:** Effect of preconditioning by four episodes of 3-minute occlusion and 5-minute reperfusion on infarct size. The control group is denoted by the solid bars, and the preconditioned group is denoted by the stippled bars. The area at risk (AR; expressed as percentage of LV weight) was similar between groups. The area of necrosis (AN; expressed as percentage of area at risk) was significantly smaller in the preconditioned group. *$p < 0.05$ vs. control. **B:** Effect of preconditioning by four episodes of 3-minute occlusion and 5-minute reperfusion on contractile function. Preconditioned hearts exhibited dyskinesis during all four episodes of 3-minute LAD occlusion and were significantly stunned just prior to the sustained 60-minute occlusion (*$p < 0.05$ vs. control). No statistically significant difference was detected between control (filled circles) and preconditioned (open circles) groups, either during the prolonged LAD occlusion or during the 4.5 hours following reflow. Base. = baseline; CO = coronary occlusion. Adapted from Ovize et al. [16] with permission of the American Heart Association.

averaged 18% of baseline values in both groups (p = NS). Thus, although preconditioning significantly reduced infarct size, it did not attenuate post-ischemic contractile dysfunction of the periinfarct tissue during the 4.5 initial hours of reflow.

Table 1. In vivo models with acute myocardial infarction

Authors (ref.)	Species	Protocol	Improved function after reflow	Comments
Ovize et al. [16]	Dog	4 × (3′ CO/5′ R) 1 h CO/4.5 h R	No	
Cohen et al. [20]	Rabbit	1 × (5′ CO/10′ R) 20′ CO/90′ R	Yes	
Ovize et al. [17]	Dog	1 × (15′ CS/10′ R) 1 h CO/4.5 h R	No	
Ovize et al. [9]	Dog	10′ stretch/10′ R 1 h CO/4.5 h R	No	
Kimura et al. [22]	Pig	4 × (5′ CO/10′ R) 1 h CO/6 h R)	Yes	Crystals in subendocardium
Ganz et al. [23]	Pig	2 × (5′ CO/5′ R) 48′ CO/30′ R	Yes	Crystals in subendocardium
Rohmann et al. [19]	Pig	1 × (10′ CO/15′ R) 1 h CO/2 h R	No	
Shizukada et al. [17]	Dog	1 × (5′ CO/10′R) (1 h CO/5 h R)	No	
Przyklenk et al. [21]	Dog	Cx: 4 × (5′ CO/5′ R) LAD: 1 h CO/4.5 h R	No[a]	

[a] Trend toward improved function in the preconditioned group due to a reduction in infarct size.
Protocol lists both the preconditioning regimen and the duration of the sustained ischemia/reperfusion.
CO = coronary occlusion; R = reperfusion; CS = coronary stenosis; Cx = circumflex coronary artery; LAD = left anterior descending coronary artery.

Subsequent studies from our laboratory and others have found a similar lack of acute improvement in postischemic contractile dysfunction with preconditioning (Table 1). For example, we found that mild ischemia (induced by partial coronary artery stenosis) is sufficient to precondition the dog heart, provided a 10-minute intervening period of complete reflow existed between the preconditioning ischemia and the subsequent prolonged coronary artery occlusion [17]. Despite a significant reduction in infarct size, recovery of postischemic contractile function was no better in preconditioned than in control hearts: At 4.5 hours after reflow, segment shortening averaged −4% vs. +3% of baseline values in preconditioned versus control groups (p = NS). Similarly, in our study of acute volume overload [9], recovery of function did not differ between preconditioned and control groups during the first 4.5 hours of reperfusion. Our results have recently been confirmed by Shizukada et al., who reported that dogs preconditioned by one episode of 5-minute coronary artery occlusion and 10 minutes of reperfusion, and then submitted to 1 hour of ischemia and 5 hours of reperfusion, did not exhibit better functional recovery [18]. In a preliminary report, Rohmann et al. also demonstrated that preconditioning did not improve postischemic contractile function in the pig heart during the first 2 hours of reflow following a 1-hour ischemic insult [19].

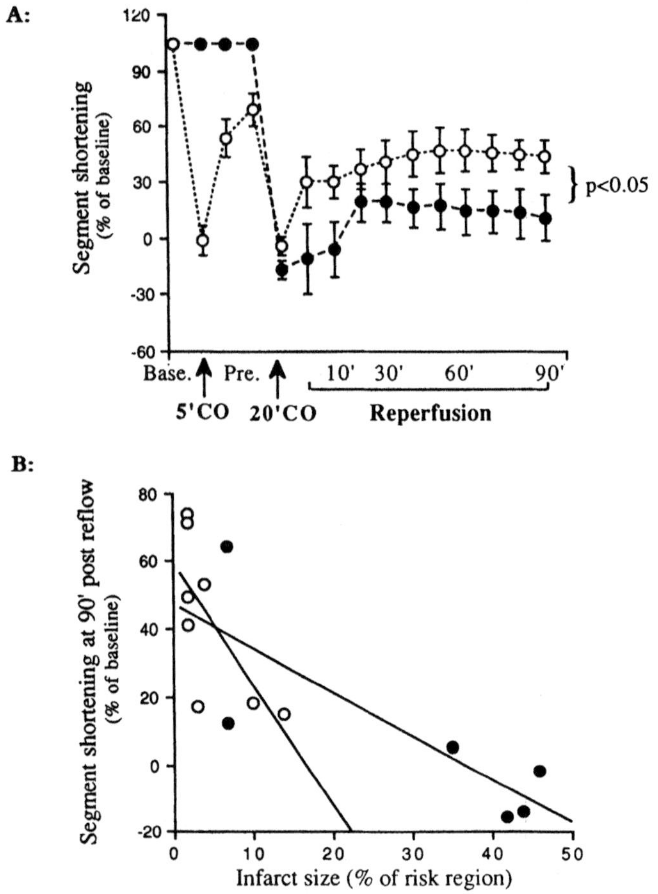

Figure 5. **A:** Segment shortening (expressed as percentage of baseline values) for control (filled circles) and preconditioned (open circles) rabbits that underwent 20 minutes of occlusion of a marginal branch of the left circumflex artery followed by 90 minutes of reflow. Recovery of function during the 90-minute period of reperfusion was significantly improved in preconditioned rabbits when compared to controls. **B:** Segment shortening at 90 minutes postreflow (expressed as percentage of baseline values) is plotted as a function of infarct size. An inverse relationship is observed for the control group (filled circles); i.e., the larger the infarct, the worse the function. A similar relationship was observed for the preconditioned group (open circles), indicating that the better functional recovery for preconditioned hearts was likely the result of infarct size reduction. Base. = baseline; CO = coronary occlusion. Reprinted from Cohen et al. [20], with permission of the American Heart Association.

In contrast, Cohen et al. have reported that preconditioning improved recovery of contractile function (assessed by sonomicrometry) during the first 90 minutes following a 20-minute coronary artery occlusion in the rabbit [20] (Figure 5A). *How can this apparent discrepancy between the rabbit and dog models be explained?* Twenty minutes of ischemia in the rabbit produces substantial necrosis, and, as a result, part of the apparent discrepancy between this work and the previously cited studies might be due to the position of ultrasonic crystals with respect to the infarcted area. Specifically, Cohen et al. positioned the crystals in the midmyocardium. Infarct size in this study averaged 29% of the myocardium at risk in control rabbits vs. 3% of the risk region in the preconditioned group [20]. This suggests that in the control animals, the crystals may have been located adjacent to (or even within) the necrotic zone, while in the preconditioned group the crystals were positioned in salvaged but stunned myocardium. Thus, the difference in segment shortening between control and preconditioned rabbits may reflect thc difference in function between necrotic myocardium vs. stunned myocardium 'tethered' to the underlying necrosis.

The confounding influence of infarct size on regional wall motion in the control and preconditioned rabbits was confirmed by plotting segment shortening as a function of infarct size [20] (Figure 5B). Not surprisingly, an inverse relationship was observed; i.e., the larger the infarct, the worse the function. If preconditioning had had an independent beneficial effect on contractile function, then data points for the preconditioned group would have been shifted upward with respect to the control regression line; i.e., better recovery of systolic function for a comparable infarct size. However, Cohen et al. found no significant difference between regression lines for the control and preconditioned groups [20]. Similar results were obtained by Przyklenk et al., who submitted dogs to 1 hour of LAD coronary artery occlusion and 4.5 hours of reperfusion [21]. In this case, the preconditioning regimen consisted of four 5-minute occlusions of a circumflex marginal branch. Preconditioned dogs developed significantly smaller infarcts than controls. There was a trend toward a better recovery of contractile function after reflow in the salvaged subepicardium of the preconditioned group (Figure 6A), but the plot of segment shortening vs. infarct size revealed that this partial effect was due to infarct size reduction (Figure 6B); that is, data points for the preconditioned group fell along the regression line for the control group, but were clustered at the "small infarct" end of the relationship. This analysis indicates that the better recovery of contractile function observed by Cohen et al. in preconditioned rabbits [20], and the trend toward improved function with "remote" preconditioning in the dog model [21], was most probably a consequence of infarct size reduction.

Two additional studies have reported that preconditioning improves the recovery of contractile function during reperfusion following the prolonged ischemic insult (Table 1). Kimura et al. submitted pig hearts to 1 hour of sustained ischemia and 6 hours of reperfusion [22]. Hearts preconditioned with four episodes of 5 minutes of coronary artery occlusion followed by 10 minutes of reflow developed significantly smaller infarcts than controls and also exhibited better recovery of postischemic contractile function. Similarly, Ganz et al. preconditioned pig hearts with two episodes of 5 minutes of

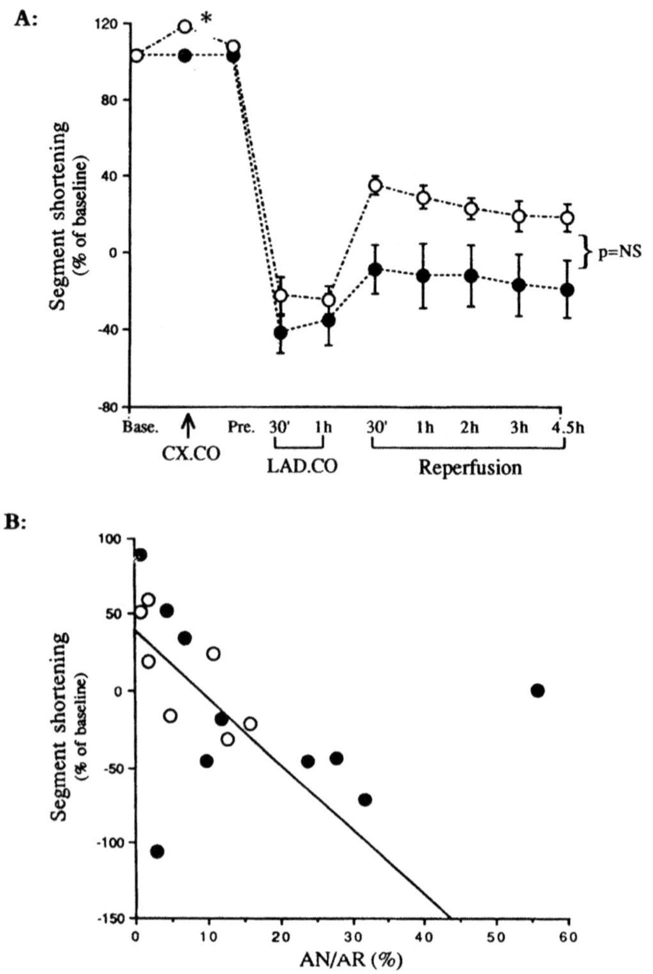

Figure 6. A: Segment shortening (expressed as percentage of baseline values) in the superficial subepicardium of the left anterior descending (LAD) coronary artery bed for control dogs (filled circles) and dogs preconditioned by four episodes of 5 minute occlusion + 5 minute reperfusion of a marginal branch of the circumflex (CX) coronary artery (open circles). CO = coronary occlusion. *$p < 0.004$ vs. baseline. **B:** Segment shortening (expressed as percentage of baseline values) measured at 4.5 hours after reperfusion and plotted as a function of infarct size. Data points for both the control (filled circles) and circumflex-preconditioned (open circles) groups fell along the same regression line. Thus, the apparent trend toward better recovery of function in the preconditioned dogs reflected the smaller infarct sizes in this group. AN = area of necrosis; AR = area at risk; Base. = baseline; Pre. = before LAD occlusion. Reprinted from Przyklenk et al. [21], with permission of the American Heart Association.

coronary artery occlusion separated by 5 minutes of reperfusion, prior to 48 minutes of ischemia followed by 30 minutes of reflow [23]. Contractile function in the preconditioned group was slightly but significantly improved during the 30-minute reperfusion period when compared with controls. Unfortunately, neither study assessed recovery of postischemic wall motion as a function of infarct size. Furthermore, in both cases, the ultrasonic crystals had been positioned in the *subendocardium* of the central ischemic zone, i.e., deep within the necrotic area. It is therefore likely that infarct size reduction played a major role in the observed benefit of preconditioning on contractile performance in these two protocols.

Thus, upon first inspection, the effect of preconditioning on postischemic contractile function after acute infarction appears controversial (Table 1): Some authors report an improvement of the recovery of contractile function during the initial hours of reflow following the prolonged ischemic insult, while others do not. However, when wall motion is analyzed as a function of infarct size, the evidence strongly suggests that improvement in function in these studies was due to infarct size reduction rather than an independent effect of preconditioning on the salvaged and stunned myocardium.

This relationship between postischemic dysfunction and extent of necrosis is complex and important. In the experiments discussed to this point, post-ischemic contractile dysfunction was due to both stunning of the viable reperfused perinecrotic tissue and tethering of this viable tissue to the necrotic subendocardium [24]. The relative contribution of stunning and tethering to this dysfunction will depend upon the extent of necrosis; When infarct size is negligible, contractile dysfunction will be exclusively due to stunning; but when infarct size is large, tethering might become more important. This distinction could be particularly relevant in these studies, since preconditioned hearts with small infarcts (i.e., mostly stunned) are being compared with control hearts (largely infarcted). This suggests that the greater the difference in infarct size between preconditioned and control groups, the higher the chance of finding a difference in the recovery of postischemic contractile function.

A second important factor that may contribute to the apparent discrepancies among studies is the duration of reperfusion following the prolonged coronary artery occlusion. In particular, the time course of stunning is dependent on both the severity and duration of the preceding ischemic insult [25]; i.e., canine myocardium stunned by 15 minutes of reversible ischemia remains impaired for hours to days following reflow, and the time required for recovery of viable subepicardium overlying subendocardial necrosis is even more prolonged [26]. Moreover, the time course of recovery of stunned myocardium may vary depending on the model that is used (rabbits vs. pigs vs. dogs). Previous preconditioning protocols have focused exclusively on *acute* recovery of wall motion. However, observation periods of less than 6 hours, particularly in the dog and pig models, may be too short to detect differences in recovery of severely stunned myocardium in a preconditioned group with negligible necrosis vs. recovery of severely stunned myocardium tethered to a large subendocardial necrosis in control animals. If the reperfusion period were prolonged to days to weeks, a difference in recovery of function between control and preconditioned groups might be unmasked. Resolution of this issue clearly awaits further investigation.

In summary, the current evidence indicates that the effects of preconditioning on acute recovery of contractile function are highly dependent on infarct size. In order to conclude that preconditioning has an independent beneficial effect on wall motion of periinfarct tissue, a significant difference in the relationship between infarct size and contractile function between control and preconditioned groups must be observed. There is no evidence to date to support this conclusion. All studies to this point have been acute (i.e., focused on the effects of preconditioning during the first 6 hours following relief of ischemia): Whether preconditioning has an independent beneficial effect on the time course of recovery of periinfarct tissue is unknown.

Does preconditioning specifically affect stunning?

Stunning is defined as the "prolonged but transient contractile dysfunction of viable myocardium that has been salvaged by reperfusion" [27]. One crucial point of the definition is that stunning refers to viable tissue. However, analysis of the specific effect of preconditioning on contractile function after prolonged coronary artery occlusion is confounded by two important factors: (1) the presence of subendocardial necrosis, which, as discussed previously, profoundly influences wall motion in the surrounding viable myocardium, and (2) the fact that the preconditioning regimen (i.e., repeated brief episodes of ischemia/reperfusion) results in contractile dysfunction before sustained ischemia, and may thereby limit or mask a beneficial effect of preconditioning on wall motion.

To address these issues, we assessed the effect of preconditioning on acute recovery of contractile function in canine myocardium stunned by a brief 15-minute ischemic insult, a duration of ischemia not associated with necrosis in the canine model [8]. We compared two different preconditioning regimens aimed at inducing tolerance to ischemia: one resulting in significant stunning before the 15-minute episode of ischemia and the other causing virtually no deterioration of contractile function. Specifically, each dog was randomly assigned to receive one of three treatments prior to the 15-minute sustained occlusion: one episode of 2.5 minutes of coronary occlusion followed by 5 minutes of reperfusion ($PC_{2.5}$ group), one episode of 5 minutes of coronary occlusion followed by 5 minutes of reperfusion (PC_5 group), or no intervention (control group). As expected, only dogs from the 5-minute-preconditioning group exhibited myocardial stunning after the brief episode of ischemia: Immediately before the 15-minute test occlusion, segment shortening averaged 101% of baseline values in the control group, 91% in the 2.5-minute

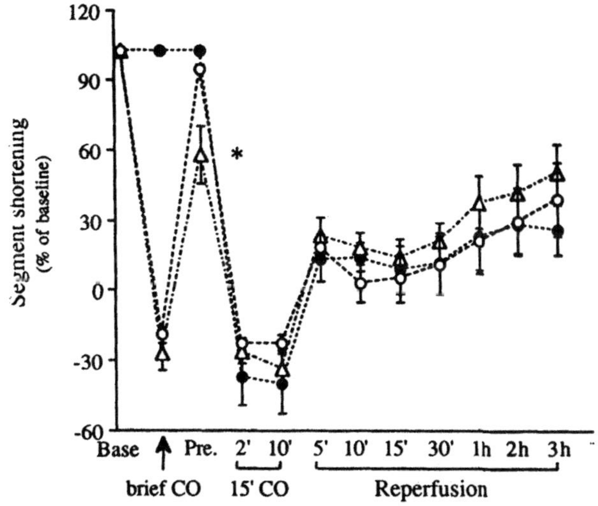

Figure 7. Effects of preconditioning on stunning. Data were obtained at baseline (Base), during the brief coronary occlusion (CO), at the end of the preconditioning phase (Pre.), and at multiple time points throughout 15 minutes of "sustained" CO and after reperfusion. Only dogs preconditioned with a 5-minute ischemia (open triangles) exhibited stunning prior to the prolonged coronary artery occlusion (*$p < 0.05$ vs. control). All groups were similarly stunned throughout the 3-hour reperfusion (control group: filled circles; PC2.5 group: open circles). Reprinted from Ovize et al. [8], with permission of the American Heart Association.

preconditioning group (p =NS vs. control), and 55% in the 5-minute preconditioning group ($p < 0.05$ vs. control; Figure 7). However, all groups demonstrated the same degree of stunning throughout reperfusion: At 3 hours after reflow, segment shortening remained depressed at 24–48% of baseline values, and did not differ significantly among the three groups (Figure 7). Segment shortening was also expressed as a function of collateral flow during coronary artery occlusion, and analysis of covariance further confirmed no significant difference among groups in the recovery of function at 3 hours after reperfusion. Thus, even an "optimal" regimen of preconditioning, which in itself does not compromise wall motion, failed to attenuate myocardial stunning during the initial hours of reperfusion in the canine model.

Similar results were recently reported by Miyamae et al., who submitted pig hearts to 15 minutes of coronary artery occlusion and 2 hours of reflow. Preconditioned hearts had previously received two episodes of 5 minutes of ischemia followed by 5 minutes of reperfusion. These authors observed that preconditioning did not attenuate stunning during the 2 hours of reperfusion (Table 2) [28]. These two studies further support the concept that preconditioning has no direct beneficial effect on acute recovery of function following more sustained ischemia/reperfusion.

Table 2. In vivo models without necrosis

Authors (Ref.)	Species	Protocol	Improved function after reflow	Comments
Ovize et al. [8]	Dog	1 × (5′ CO/5′ R)	No	No necrosis
Miyamae et al. [28]	Pig	2 × (5′ CO/5′ R) 15′ CO/2 h R	No	No necrosis

Protocol lists both the preconditioning regimen and the duration of the sustained ischemia/reperfusion.
CO = coronary occlusion; R = reperfusion.

EFFECT OF PRECONDITIONING ON CONTRACTILE FUNCTION IN ISOLATED PERFUSED HEART PREPARATIONS

In isolated perfused heart preparations, the preconditioning regimen typically consists of one or more episodes of 5 minutes of global ischemia or hypoxia. Then, isolated hearts usually undergo a 30- to 60-minute period of sustained global ischemia followed by 30–60 minutes of reperfusion. Contractile function after reflow is assessed by measurement of left ventricle developed pressure, rate-pressure product, or dP/dt. Interestingly, in contrast to in vivo studies, all isolated heart studies have reported a beneficial effect of preconditioning on recovery of contractile function during reperfusion (Table 3).

How to explain this discrepancy between in vivo and ex vivo studies?

Several studies have clearly demonstrated that isolated perfused rat or rabbit hearts are reversibly injured by a brief 5- or 10-minute period of global ischemia [30–32]. In other words, isolated rat and rabbit hearts appear to exhibit "stunning" after a brief nonlethal ischemic episode. However, *stunned myocardium* by definition implies that contractile function will eventually be restored to normal baseline values. But, recovery of normal contractile function after a brief reversible ischemic insult may take hours or even days [30], a period of time beyond the scope of the isolated perfused heart (and open-chest in-situ) preparations. Consequently, the only way to determine whether these preparations represent true models of stunning is to ensure that no irreversible damage occurred as a result of the ischemic insult. Evidence of the absence of irreversible damage can be obtained either directly (i.e., macroscopic staining or electron microscopy) or indirectly (i.e., by assessing the response of the heart to inotropic stimulation, or by determining whether resumption of oxidative phosphorylation has occurred). In any case, any conclusion that preconditioning (or any other intervention) favorably affects stunning requires evidence of either full recovery of postischemic contractile function, or absence of irreversible cellular damage, in the model under study. There is currently no study reporting the effect of preconditioning on contractile function after a purely *reversible* ischemic insult in the isolated perfused heart.

Table 3. Isolated heart studies

Authors (Ref.)	Species	Protocol	Improved function after reflow	Comments
Omar et al. [36]	Rabbit	1 × (5′ isch/5′ R) 1 h isch/1 h R	Yes	
Barakat et al. [39]	Rat	1 × (5′ isch/10′ R) 30′ isch/45′ R	Yes	No quantitation of cellular injury
Lasley et al. [37]	Rat	1 × (5′ isch/10′ R) 30′ isch/30′ R	Yes	No quantitation of cellular injury
Hendrikx et al. [38]	Rabbit	1 × (5′ isch/5′ R) 45′ isch/1 h R	Yes	No quantitation of cellular injury
Asimakis et al. [34]	Rat	1 or 2 × (5′ isch/5′ R) 40′ isch/30′ R	Yes	No quantitation of cellular injury
Grover et al. [35]	Rat	4 × (5′ isch/5′ R) 30′ isch/30′ R	Yes	

Protocol lists both the preconditioning regimen and the duration of the sustained ischemia/reperfusion.
isch = ischemia; R = reperfusion.

All published preconditioning studies performed in the isolated perfused heart preparation have used durations of global ischemia (or hypoxia) ranging from 30 to 60 minutes (Table 3). It is well established that in this preparation, such prolonged periods of ischemia result in substantial irreversible damage. For example, after 30 minutes of ischemia in the isolated rabbit heart, Borgers et al. reported that 80% of subendocardial myocytes and 60% of subepicardial myocytes exhibit cytolysis, pyknolysis of nuclei, and contraction band necrosis [33]. Similarly, the proportion of rat myocytes that are still viable following ≥30 minutes of global ischemia/reperfusion is small [31]. Moreover, prolonged (>10 minute) periods of global ischemia result in massive calcium overload upon reperfusion and profound diastolic contracture—a further indicator of irreversible tissue injury [34]. In other words, 30 minutes of global ischemia followed by reperfusion in isolated perfused rat or rabbit hearts does not represent a *"pure" model of stunning*. This is in agreement with a preliminary study of Grover et al., who showed significant release of lactate dehydrogenase (LDH; an index of irreversible cellular injury) in both control and preconditioned rat hearts after a 30-minute period of normothermic ischemia followed by 30 minutes of reflow [35]. Similarly, Omar et al. observed significant release of LDH in the coronary effluent in both control and preconditioned rabbit hearts after 1 hour of ischemia and 1 hour of reperfusion [36] (Figure 8). In both studies, preconditioning both reduced the release of enzyme (i.e., reduced the severity of irreversible injury) and improved postischemic recovery of LV developed pressure. Other preconditioning studies, using similar isolated heart preparations, have also observed significant improvement of postischemic contractile function asso-

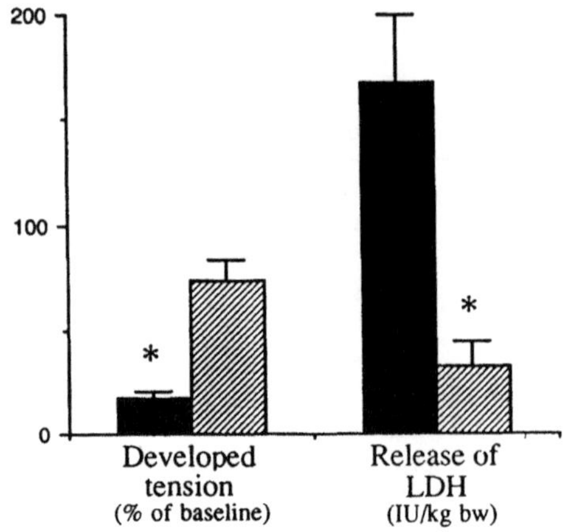

Figure 8. Effects of preconditioning on left ventricular (LV) developed tension and release of lactate dehydrogenase (LDH) from isolated rabbit hearts. Preconditioning significantly improved developed tension during reperfusion and markedly reduced LDH release (*$p < 0.05$) following 60 minutes of global ischemia. This suggests that better functional recovery in preconditioned isolated rabbit hearts was a consequence of myocyte salvage. Solid bars denote the control group; hatched bars denote the preconditioned group. Adapted with permission from Omar et al. [36].

ciated with preconditioning but, unfortunately, cellular integrity was not assessed [37–39]. In order to determine whether improvement in contractile performance with preconditioning in the isolated heart preparations is dependent or independent of myocyte salvage, developed pressure (or any other index of contractile function) should be expressed as a function of LDH release (or other indices of tissue injury).

In summary, it is likely that better recovery of contractile function associated with preconditioning in the isolated perfused heart models may reflect a preservation of myocyte viability (i.e., a "reduction in infarct size"). Whether, in the isolated heart model, preconditioning truly affects stunning resulting from reversible ischemia remains to be determined.

CONCLUSIONS

There is now sufficient evidence to conclusively state that preconditioning is not a consequence of myocardial stunning. The time course and severity of the two phenomena can be dissociated, and preconditioning can, in fact, be induced in the absence of previous stunning. The effects of preconditioning on the acute recovery of contractile function after an irreversible ischemic insult are complex and are likely dependent upon infarct size reduction. There is currently no evidence that preconditioning exerts a direct beneficial effect on contractile function of reversibly injured myocardium during the initial hours following relief of ischemia.

REFERENCES

1. Murry CE, Jennings RB, Reimer KA. 1986. Preconditioning with ischemia: A delay of lethal cell injury in ischemic myocardium. Circulation 5:1124–1136.
2. Murry CE, Richard V, Reimer KA, Jennings RB 1990. Ischemic preconditioning slows energy metabolism and delays ultrastructural damage during a sustained ischemic episode. Circ Res 66:913–931.
3. Murry CE, Richard V, Jennings RB, Reimer KA. 1991. Myocardial protection is lost before contractile function recovers from ischemic preconditioning. Am J Physiol 260:H796–H804.
4. Schröder E, Kieso RA, Laughlin D, Schröder M, Meng R, Kerber RE. 1987. Altered response of reperfused myocardium to repeated coronary occlusion in dogs. J Am Coll Cardiol 19:898–905.
5. Miura T, Goto M, Urabe K, Endoch A, Shimamoto K, Iimura O. 1991. Does myocardial stunning contribute to infarct size limitation by ischemic preconditioning? Circulation 84:2504–2512.
6. Hale SL, Kloner RA. 1992. Effect of ischemic preconditioning on regional myocardial blood flow in the rabbit heart. Coronary Artery Dis 3:133–140.
7. Li GC, Vasquez JA, Gallagher KP, Lucchesi BR. 1990. Myocardial protection with preconditioning. Circulation 82:609–619.
8. Ovize M, Przyklenk K, Kloner RA. 1992. Preconditioning does not attenuate myocardial stunning. Circulation 85:2247–2254.
9. Ovize M, Kloner RA, Przyklenk K. 1992. Myocardial dilation, in the absence of ischemia, preconditions the canine myocardium. Circulation 86:I32 (abstr).
10. Rohmann S, Schott RJ, Harting J, Schaper W. 1991. Ischemic preconditioning is not a function of stunned myocardium. J Mol Cell Cardio 23:S71 (abstr).
11. Liu GS, Thornton J, Van Winkle DM, Stanley AWH, Olsson RA, Downey JM. 1991. Protection against infarction afforded by preconditioning is mediated by A_1 adenosine receptors in rabbit heart. Circulation 84:350–356.
12. Gross GJ, Auchampach JA. 1992. Blockade of ATP-sensitive potassium channels prevents myocardial preconditioning in dogs. Circ Res 70:223–233.
13. Shiki K, Hearse DJ. 1987. Preconditioning of ischemic myocardium: Reperfusion-induced arrhythmias. Am J Physiol 253:H1470–1476.
14. Hagar JM, Hale SL, Kloner RA. 1991. Effect of preconditioning ischemia on reperfusion arrhythmias after coronary artery occlusion and reperfusion in the rat. Circ Res 68:61–68.
15. Li Y, Whittaker P, Kloner RA. 1992. The transient nature of the effect of ischemic preconditioning on myocardial infarct size and ventricular arrythmia. Am Heart J 123: 346–353.
16. Ovize M, Kloner RA, Hale SL, Przyklenk K. 1992. Coronary cyclic flow variations precondition the ischemic myocardium. Circulation 85:779–789.
17. Ovize M, Przyklenk K, Kloner RA. 1992. Partial stenosis is sufficient and complete reperfusion is mandatory for preconditioning the canine heart. Circ Res 71:1165–1173
18. Shizukada Y, Mallet RT, Lee Sc, Downey HF. 1992. Hypoxic preconditioning of ischemic canine myocardium. Cardiovasc Res 26:534–542.
19. Rohmann S, Weygandt H, Schelling P, Lues I, Merck E. 1992. ATP-sensitive potassium channel opener bimakalim mimics preconditioning protection in swine. Circulation 86:I555 (abstr).
20. Cohen MV, Liu GS, Downey JM. 1991. Preconditioning causes improved wall motion as well as smaller infarcts after transient coronary occlusion in rabbits. Circulation 84:341–349.
21. Przyklenk K, Bauer B, Ovize M, Kloner RA, Whittaker P. 1993. Regional ischemic preconditioning protects remote virgin myocardium from subsequent coronary occlusion. Circulation 87:893–899.
22. Kimura Y, Iyengar J, Subramanian R, Cordis GA, Das DK. 1992. Preconditioning of the heart by repeated stunning: Attenuation of postischemic dysfunction. Basic Res Cardiol 87:128–138.
23. Ganz E, Garcia-Dorado D, Oliveras J, Perez-Villa F, Carreras MJ, Théroux P, Soler-Soler J. 1992. Ischemic preconditioning limits post-reperfusion myocardial edema and preserves left ventricular function. J Am Coll Cardiol 19:118A (abstr).
24. Weintraub WS, Hattori S, Agarwall JB, Bodenheimer MM, Banka VS, Helfant RH. 1981.

The relationship between myocardial blood flow and contraction by myocardial layer in the canine left ventricle during ischemia. Circ Res 48:430–438.
25. Bolli R, Zhu WX, Thornby JI, O'Neill PG, Roberts R. 1988. Time course and determinants of recovery of function after reversible ischemia in conscious dogs. Am J Physiol 254: H102–H114.
26. Ellis SG, Henschke CI, Sandor T, Wynne J, Braunwald E, Kloner RA. 1983. Time course of functional and biochemical recovery of myocardium salvaged by reperfusion. J Am Coll Cardiol 1:1047–1055.
27. Braunwald E, Kloner RA. 1992. The stunned myocardium: Prolonged, postischemic ventricular dysfunction. Circulation 66:1146–1149.
28. Miyamae M, Fujiwara H, Yokota R, Kida M, Katsuragawa M, Tanaka M, Ohura M, Yabuuchi Y. 1992. Ischemic preconditioning accelerates energy production but does not improve stunning in porcine hearts. Circulation 86:I339 (abstr).
29. Heyndrickx GR, Millard RW, McRitchie RJ, Maroko PR, Vatner SF. 1975. Regional myocardial functional and electrophysiological alterations after brief coronary artery occlusion in conscious dogs. J Clin Invest 56:978–985.
30. Apstein CS, Deckelbaum L, Hagopian L, Hood W. 1978. Acute cardiac ischemia and reperfusion: Contractility, relaxation, and glycolysis. Am J Physiol 235:H637.
31. Nayler WG, Elz JS, Buckley DJ. 1988. The stunned myocardium: Effects of electrical and mechanical arrest and osmolarity. Am J Physiol 254:H60.
32. Nayler WG, Liu J, Panagiotopoulos S. 1990. Nifedipine and experimental cardioprotection. Cardiovasc Drugs Ther 4:879–886.
33. Borgers M, Shu LG, Xhonneux R, Thone F, van Overloop P. 1987. Changes in ultrastructure and Ca^{++} distribution in the isolated working rabbit heart after ischemia: A time-related study. Am J Pathol 126:92–102.
34. Asimakis GK, Inners-McBride K, Medellen G, Conti VR. 1992. Ischemic preconditioning attenuates acidosis and postischemic dysfunction in isolated rat heart. Am J Physiol 263: H887–H894.
35. Grover GJ, Dzwonczyk S, Sleph PG. 1992. ATP-sensitive K^+ channel activation does not mediate preconditioning in isolated rat hearts. Circulation 86:I342 (abstr).
36. Omar BA, Hanson AK, Bose SK, McCord JM. 1991. Reperfusion with pyruvate eliminates ischemic preconditioning in the isolated rabbit heart: An apparent role for enhanced glycolysis. Coronary Artery Dis 2:799–804.
37. Lasley RD, Anderson GM, Mentzer RM, Jr. 1992. Adenosine receptor blockade does not block hypoxic preconditioning in the isolated rat heart. Circulation 86:I342 (abstr).
38. Hendrikx M, Toshima Y, Mubagwa K, Flameng W. 1992. Improved functional recovery after ischemic preconditioning in the globally ischemic rabbit heart is not mediated by adenosine A1 receptor activation. Circulation 86:I342 (abstr).
39. Barakat O, van Wylen DGL, Mehtzer RM, Jr, Lasley RD. 1991. Ischemic preconditioning improves postischemic recovery of function but shortens time to onset of ischemic contracture in isolated rat hearts. Circulation 84:II433 (abstr).

4. PRECONDITIONING AND THE CORONARY VASCULATURE

BARBARA BAUER, ROBERT A. KLONER, and KARIN PRZYKLENK

INTRODUCTION

In 1986, Murry et al. showed that repeated short episodes of coronary occlusion protect the myocytes against subsequent sustained ischemia: This phenomenon was termed *ischemic preconditioning* [1]. While there is no doubt that preconditioning limits infarct size, myocardial necrosis is not the only consequence of sustained/ischemia reperfusion: One or more hours of occlusion followed by reflow also results in ventricular arrhythmias, postischemic contractile dysfunction or "stunning," and abnormalities in myocardial perfusion. The obvious question therefore arises: Do the benefits of ischemic preconditioning extend beyond the concept of myocyte viability and attenuate other deleterious sequelae associated with sustained ischemia/reperfusion?

In this chapter, we focus on the coronary vasculature, and possible protective effects of preconditioning on the *loss of coronary vasodilator reserve* and the *"low-reflow" phenomenon* as deleterious consequences of myocardial ischemia/reperfusion.

ISCHEMIA/REPERFUSION INJURY EXTENDS TO THE CORONARY VASCULATURE

Loss in coronary vasodilator reserve

Sustained ischemia/reperfusion results in a loss in coronary vasodilator reserve: This has been extensively documented in both isolated arterial rings

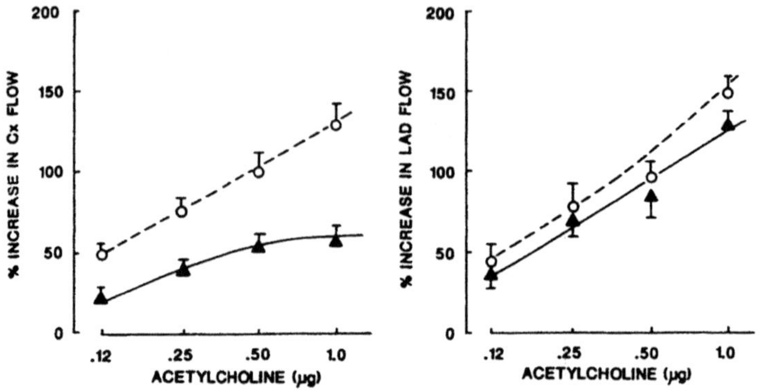

Figure 1. Percent increase in circumflex (Cx) and left anterior descending (LAD) coronary blood flow in response to acetylcholine (0.12–1.0 μg intracoronary), administered at baseline (open circles) and following 1 hour of Cx occlusion/reperfusion (filled triangles) in the in vivo canine model. A decrease in the response to acetylcholine was observed in the ischemic/reperfused Cx bed ($p < 0.01$ vs. baseline), but not in the LAD bed. Reprinted with permission from Mehta et al. [4].

previously exposed to ischemia [2,3] and in vivo models of coronary artery occlusion followed by reperfusion [4]. For example, Mehta et al. [4] showed in anesthetized dogs that the increase in blood flow in response to the vasodilators acetylcholine and bradykinin was significantly impaired by 1 hour of total coronary occlusion and 1 hour of reperfusion (Figure 1).

Furchgott et al. [5] first described the obligatory role of the endothelium in the regulation of vascular tone to a variety of vasodilators. Recently, attention has focused on the role of the endothelium in ischemia-reperfusion injury, as damage to the endothelium or development of endothelial dysfunction may impair release of vasoactive substances such as endothelium-derived relaxing factor (EDRF) [6]. In addition, endothelial generation of superoxide radicals may act as a trigger mechanism for endothelial dysfunction during reperfusion, which is then amplified by neutrophil adherence and diapedesis into the ischemic region, thereby enhancing postreperfusion ischemic injury [7].

"No reflow" and "low reflow"

The no-reflow phenomenon is defined as the inability to reperfuse previously ischemic myocardium [8]. No-reflow, which has been shown to worsen as a function of time following reperfusion, is most likely due to microvascular damage, perhaps mediated by oxygen free radicals [9,10]. Neutrophil plugs also have been suggested as a possible cause for no reflow [11]. Evidence obtained in the canine model indicates that no reflow is characterized by a severe reduction in myocardial blood flow to less than 35% of baseline values, is seen only following prolonged (≥1 hour) episodes of sustained coronary occlusion, and occurs only within regions of necrotic myocardium [12,13].

In contrast, low reflow is characterized by a mild depression in blood flow (i.e., averaging 60–85% of normal values) in viable, previously ischemic myocardium that has been salvaged by reperfusion. Even a 15-minute period of sustained ischemia can result in subsequent mild low reflow, and, as was the case with no reflow, the severity of low reflow appears to worsen during the initial hours following reperfusion [12,14]. Low reflow is not, however, caused by gross morphologic injury to the coronary vasculature, and the etiology of this phenomenon remains uncertain [15].

RATIONALE FOR A POSSIBLE BENEFIT OF PRECONDITIONING ON THE CORONARY VASCULATURE

Several studies have shown that adenosine receptor antagonists can attenuate or even abolish the reduction in infarct size achieved with preconditioning, suggesting that preconditioning may be mediated by release of adenosine and activation of cardiac A_1 receptors [16,17]. Adenosine is rapidly taken up by endothelial cells and is known to be a potent endogenous arteriolar vasodilator [18]. It has been shown to reduce neutrophil-mediated endothelial damage, thereby preserving endothelial cell structure in the ischemic zone and preventing the progressive decrease in microcirculatory flow [19]. Thus a possible preservation of endothelial function mediated by release of adenosine during "preconditioning" might contribute to the mechanism of myocardial salvage, and might attenuate low reflow and the loss in vasodilator reserve following sustained occlusion/reperfusion.

PRECONDITIONING AND CORONARY VASODILATOR RESERVE

We addressed the issue of preconditioning and loss of vasodilator reserve in the anesthetized open-chest canine model [20]. Dogs were randomly assigned to undergo either brief preconditioning ischemia (i.e., four episodes of 5 minutes coronary occlusion + 5 minutes reperfusion) or no intervention prior to 1 hour of sustained coronary artery occlusion and 4 hours of reflow. Endothelium-dependent vasodilator reserve was assessed repeatedly during the protocol by monitoring the increase in coronary blood flow in response to acetylcholine (0.01 mg administered intravenously).

We found that both control and preconditioned dogs exhibited a loss in endothelium-dependent vasodilator reserve between 30 minutes and 4 hours postreperfusion (Figures 2 and 3). Specifically, coronary blood flow in response to acetylcholine challenge increased to approximately 175–200% of baseline values before occlusion, remained essentially unchanged at 30 minutes following reflow, but increased to only 130–160% of baseline at 4 hours following relief of ischemia. We found no difference in the response to

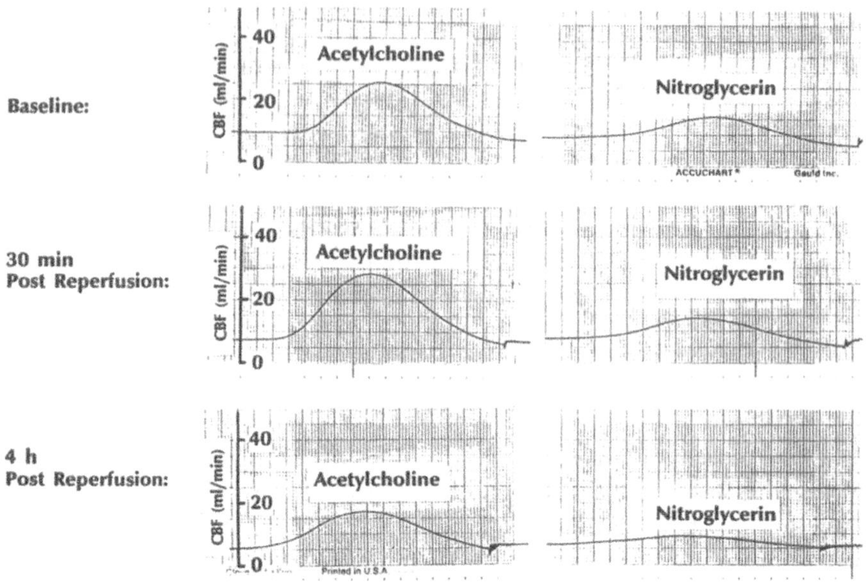

Figure 2. Representative recording of the change in coronary blood flow in response to acetylcholine (0.01 mg intravenous) and nitroglycerin (0.05 mg intravenous), assessed at baseline and at 30 minutes and 4 hours after reperfusion, for one control dog in the study. The vasodilator response to both agents did not change between baseline and 30 minutes after reperfusion, but decreased during the subsequent 3.5 hours of reflow. CBF = coronary blood flow. Reprinted with permission from Bauer et al. [20].

acetylcholine between control and preconditioned groups (Figure 3). We also observed a decrease in the response to the endothelium-independent vasodilator nitroglycerin (0.05 mg intravenously) in both control and preconditioned groups (Figures 2 and 3), probably reflecting dysfunction of the vascular smooth muscle and/or reduction in cross-sectional area of the coronary vascular bed by neutrophil plugging or by myocyte or endothelial edema [21]. Most importantly, the response to acetylcholine and nitroglycerin did not differ between the control and the preconditioned groups at any time during the experiment. Thus, preconditioning did not protect against the deterioration in coronary vasodilator reserve following sustained ischemia/reperfusion in this canine model.

Only two other reports have specifically focused on the effects of ischemic preconditioning on coronary vasodilation [22,23]. In anesthetized open-chest dogs, coronary arteriolar diameters in the in vivo beating heart were determined by intravital microscopy during intracoronary infusion of the endothelium-dependent agonist serotonin. The serotonin-induced increase in arteriolar diameter observed in control dogs (9.0 ± 3.8%) was significantly attenuated after 60 minutes of ischemia and 90 minutes of reperfusion (0.8

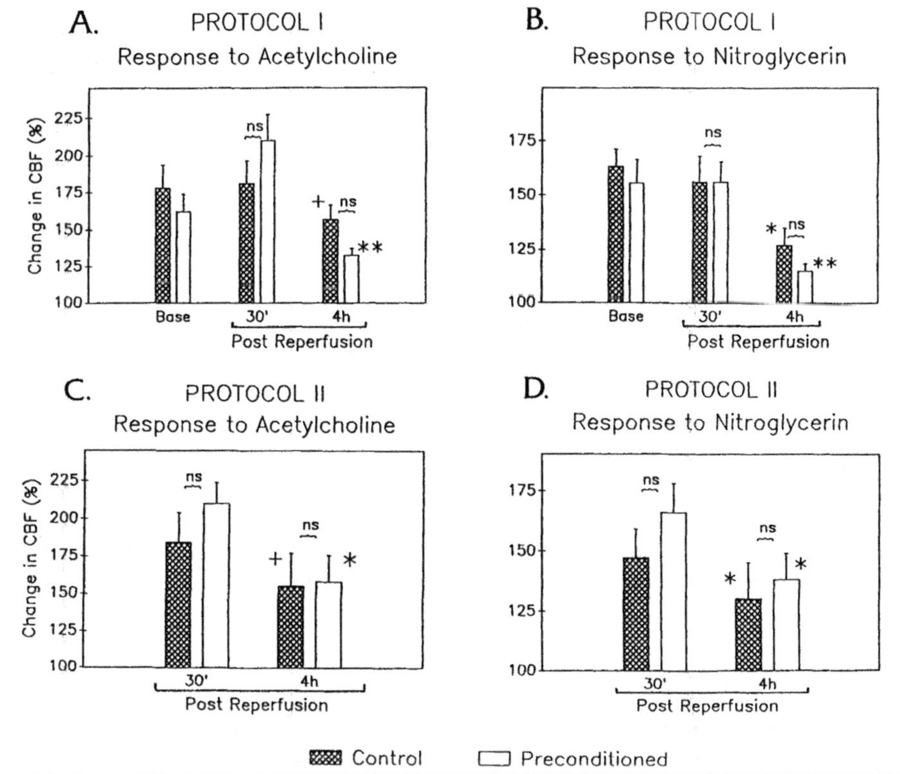

Figure 3. Change in coronary blood flow in response to acetylcholine and nitroglycerin, expressed as the maximum percent increase in coronary blood flow with respect to baseline values measured at the beginning of each experiment. In Protocol I **(A,B)**, acetylcholine and nitroglycerin were administered at baseline and at 30 minutes and 4 hours after reperfusion. In contrast, in Protocol II **(C,D)**, vasodilators were only administered after reperfusion in order to avoid an apparent cardioprotective effect of these agents when given before occlusion. In both Protocols, the vasodilator response to both acetylcholine and nitroglycerin deteriorated between 30 minutes and 4 hours postreperfusion, with no difference between control and preconditioned groups. CBF = coronary blood flow; Base = baseline.

± 2.0%; $p < 0.05$). However, in dogs preconditioned with a single 10-minute brief coronary occlusion, serotonin-mediated dilation was preserved (7.6 ± 3.1%; Figure 4). These authors have recently expanded upon this preliminary observation and have reported that preconditioning also preserves acetylcholine-mediated increases in coronary arteriolar diameter [23].

Reasons for the apparent discrepancy between the studies are uncertain. Obvious differences in the choice of the preconditioning regimen or in the method used to assess coronary vasodilator reserve might be possible explanations. Furthermore, in our study *maximal* coronary vasodilator reserve was not assessed: Differences between control and preconditioned animals may have become apparent at maximal vasodilation.

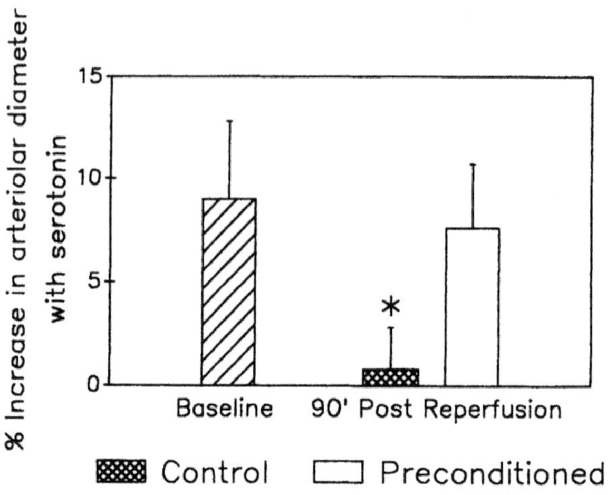

Figure 4. Percent increase in coronary arteriolar diameter with serotonin challenge in the in vivo dog model. After 1 hour of sustained coronary occlusion and 90 minutes of reperfusion, the vasodilator response to serotonin was significantly impaired in control dogs, but was preserved in preconditioned animals. Adapted with permission from DeFily et al. [22].

It could be questioned whether the preconditioning regimen per se compromised vascular reactivity and thus confounded the premise of our study. In previous studies, neither 12 repeated episodes of 5 minutes coronary occlusion + 10 minutes reperfusion, nor three episodes of 10 minutes occlusion + 30 minutes reperfusion impaired coronary vasodilator reserve during subsequent sustained reperfusion [24,25]. In addition, evidence from our laboratory indicates that our specific preconditioning stimulus (four episodes of 5 minutes occlusion + 5 minutes reperfusion) had no effect on the subsequent response to acetylcholine or nitroglycerin [20]. These results indicate that repeated short (≤10-minute) episodes of transient ischemia interrupted by transient reflow used to precondition the myocardium do not appear to impair vasodilator reserve.

PRECONDITIONING AND THE NO/LOW-REFLOW PHENOMENA

In addition to the loss in vasodilator reserve observed in all dogs in our study, both preconditioned and control groups exhibited a significant deterioration in resting myocardial perfusion (assessed by repeated injection of radiolabelled microspheres) following relief of ischemia [20]. For example, in Protocol II, blood flow to the previously ischemic subendocardium measured at 30 minutes and 4 hours following reperfusion decreased from 1.84 to 0.55 ml/min/g tissue in control animals, and from 0.74 to 0.50 ml/min/g in the preconditioned group(Figure 5 C). Deterioration in blood flow, albeit less pronounced, was also observed in the previously ischemic subepicardium.

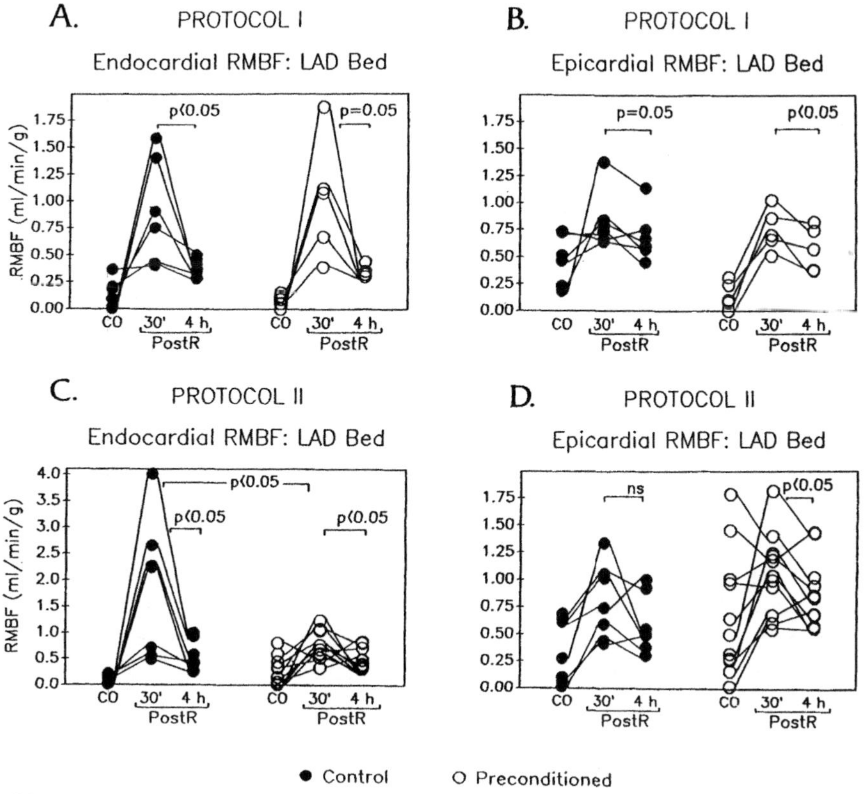

Figure 5. Regional myocardial blood flow (RMBF: ml/min/g tissue) in the ischemic/reperfused left anterior descending (LAD) coronary artery bed, measured by injection of radiolabeled microspheres, for each dog in Protocol I (**A,B**; dilators given at baseline and after reperfusion) and protocol II (**C,D**; dilators given only after reperfusion). Endocardial and epicardial values were measured during sustained LAD occlusion and at 30 minutes and 4 hours following reperfusion. Low reflow was observed in both protocols (i.e., myocardial blood flow deteriorated between 30 minutes and 4 hours postreperfusion), and this deterioration in resting myocardial perfusion was not prevented by preconditioning. However, in Protocol II, subendocardial blood flow at 30 minutes after reperfusion was significantly *lower* in preconditioned animals than in the control group. CO = coronary artery occlusion; R = reperfusion; ns = difference not significant. Reprinted with permission from Bauer et al. [20].

The extent of infarction, determined by triphenyltetrazolium staining, was confined to the subendocardium in all dogs. Thus, the decrease in subepicardial flow involved only viable tissue (and was, by definition low reflow), whereas the deterioration in flow in the ischemic/reperfused subendocardium may represent a mixture of both no reflow (i.e., an anatomic perfusion defect within the subendocardial necrosis) and low reflow in the remaining viable tissue. Most importantly, our results indicate that *preconditioning did not prevent the decrease in resting perfusion in either the sub-*

epicardium (i.e., did not prevent low reflow) or subendocardium (mixture of low reflow and no reflow) observed at 4 hours following reflow in this canine model [20].

Other studies, performed in the in vivo dog and pig model, are in agreement with our results: In the ischemic-reperfused region, there was no significant difference in regional myocardial blood flow between preconditioned and control animals measured at 25 minutes [26], 3 hours [27], or 5 hours [28] during reperfusion.

In apparent contrast to these data, Hale and Kloner [29] report that, after 40 minutes of coronary occlusion and 3 hours of reperfusion in the rabbit model, flow to the previously ischemic myocardium was significantly higher in preconditioned hearts than in controls (Figure 6). How can this difference between the two models be explained? The answer may lie in the differences in the volume of infarcted myocardium (and thus the volume of myocardium susceptible to no reflow) in the two preparations, rather than a difference in the effects of preconditioning on the vasculature per se. Specifically, infarct sizes in the rabbit model were large, averaging 53% and 30% of the myocardium at risk in control and preconditioned groups [29]. In addition, the infarcts in both groups of rabbits involved the subendocardial, midmyocardial and subepicardial layers. This 23% reduction in the transmural extent of infarction (and the corresponding 23% reduction in the probable extent of no reflow) may account for the higher values of transmural blood flow following reperfusion in the preconditioned group than in controls (0.91 ± 0.11 vs. 0.61 ± 0.09 ml/min/g tissue, respectively). However, even in

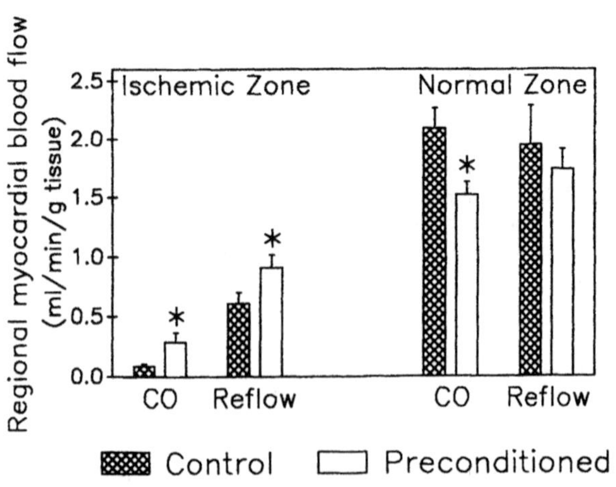

Figure 6. Regional myocardial blood flow (RMBF) measured during sustained occlusion and at 3 hours after reperfusion in the in vivo rabbit model. RMBF in the ischemic/reperfused zone was significantly higher at 3 hours following reflow in preconditioned rabbits when compared with controls. CO = coronary artery occlusion; *p < 0.05 vs. control. Adapted with permission from Hale et al. [25].

preconditioned rabbits, blood flow following reperfusion remained substantially lower than the values of 1.5–2 ml/min/g observed in normally perfused regions of the heart [29]. Thus, salvaged myocardium in the ischemic/reperfused territory exhibited low reflow. In contrast, in our dog model, infarct size was 11% and 2% of the myocardium at risk in the control and preconditioned groups [20], respectively. This more modest difference in the extent of infarction, combined with the patchy subendocardial nature of the necrosis in this model, may have precluded the detection of a possible difference in resting subendocardial blood flow between control and preconditioned dogs.

SECONDARY OBSERVATIONS: CLUES CONCERNING THE MECHANISM(S) OF PRECONDITIONING?

Acetylcholine mimics the protective effect of preconditioning?

An important secondary observation that arose from our protocol was that when the vasodilators acetylcholine and nitroglycerin were injected prior to sustained occlusion, even the most severely ischemic control dogs had significantly smaller infarcts after 1 hour of LAD occlusion when compared with control animals not pretreated with the dilators [20]. Thus, the vasodilators seemed to reduce infarct size to a similar extent as that achieved by preconditioning (Figure 7).

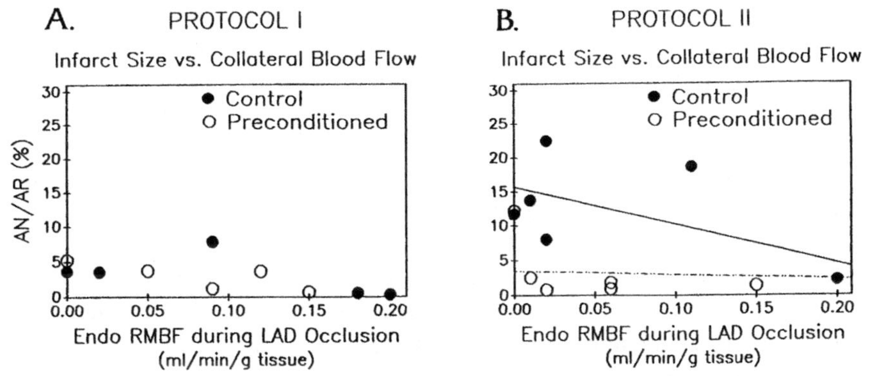

Figure 7. Infarct size plotted as a function of collateral blood flow for dogs in Protocol I (**A**; dilators given at baseline and after reperfusion) and Protocol II (**B**; dilators given only after reperfusion). In Protocol I, all dogs developed small infarcts; i.e., even the most severely ischemic control dogs appeared to have been preconditioned. In Protocol II, however, preconditioning resulted in the expected reduction in infarct size for all levels of collateral perfusion ($F = 9.39$ and $p < 0.05$ vs. controls by analysis of covariance). AN = area of necrosis; AR = area at risk; Endo RMBF = regional myocardial blood flow in the subendocardium; LAD = left anterior descending coronary artery. Reprinted with permission from Bauer et al. [20].

The explanation for this cardioprotection conferred by the vasodilators is unresolved. The bolus injection of nitroglycerin given before ischemia was probably not responsible for this reduction in infarct size in control animals, as the half-life of this agent is only on the order of 3 minutes. However, injections of both acetylcholine and nitroglycerin obviously evoked alterations in coronary blood flow (see Figure 2). Cyclic flow variations resulting in transient (but severe) episodes of myocardial ischemia have been shown to precondition the canine heart [27], but whether the smaller amplitude of flow variation produced by the dilators is sufficient to induce the cardioprotective effect is unknown. Perhaps the most likely explanation involves the possible consequences of acetylcholine pretreatment. Acetylcholine administered before sustained ischemia has recently been reported to be as effective as ischemic preconditioning or adenosine receptor agonists in protecting hearts from infarction in the rabbit model [30]. Activation of the G_i protein, coupled with the muscarinic cholinergic receptor as well as with the A_1 receptor, might be responsible for the protection [30]. Whether this might also account for the preconditioning effect of the vasodilators injected prior to sustained coronary occlusion in our canine model is the subject of ongoing investigation.

Preconditioning blunts reactive hyperemia following relief of sustained ischemia

A further unexpected observation in our study [20] was that in animals in which the dilators were given only after reperfusion (i.e., animals that were not preconditioned by administration of acetylcholine and/or nitroglycerin before sustained ischemia), subendocardial blood flow measured at 30 minutes after reflow was significantly *lower* in preconditioned dogs than in controls (Figure 5). As reactive hyperemia has been attributed, at least in part, to accumulation of adenosine during coronary occlusion and subsequent washout upon reperfusion [15,21], these data suggest that the washout of adenosine might be attenuated in preconditioned dogs vs. controls. However, Kitakaze and colleagues [31] have reported the converse; i.e., adenosine release was significantly *higher* in preconditioned dogs than in controls throughout the initial 40 minutes following relief of sustained ischemia. The results from our study, combined with the enhanced adenosine levels measured by Kitakaze et al. [30], may indicate that the sensitivity of the coronary vasculature to adenosine, but not acetylcholine, is reduced by preconditioning. This hypothesis, however, remains to be tested.

SUMMARY

There is no doubt that ischemic preconditioning protects the myocytes from a subsequent 1 hour episode of coronary occlusion by an as-yet unknown mechanism. In contrast, the effects of preconditioning on the coronary vasculature remain less well defined. While there is some evidence for improved myocardial perfusion following relief of ischemia in the in vivo rabbit model, this is probably a secondary consequence of myocardial protection (i.e., reduction in no reflow due to salvage of large volumes of ischemic myocardium) rather than a direct effect of preconditioning on the vasculature. However, in the anesthetized canine model, preconditioning neither prevents the detoriation in resting myocardial blood flow nor blunts the loss in vasodilator reserve observed during the initial hours following relief of sustained ischemia.

ACKNOWLEDGMENT

The authors thank Christl Wolff for typing the manuscript.

REFERENCES

1. Murry CE, Jennings RB, Reimer KA. 1986. Preconditioning with ischemia: A delay of lethal cell injury in ischemic myocardium. Circulation 74:1124–1136.
2. Ku DD. 1982. Coronary vascular reactivity after acute myocardial ischmia. Science 218: 576–578.
3. Van Benthuysen KM, McMurry IF, Horowitz LD. 1987. Reperfusion after acute coronary occlusion in dogs impairs endothelium-dependent relaxation to acetylcholine and augments contractile reactivity in vivo. J Clin Invest 79:265–274.
4. Mehta JL, Nichols WW, Donnelly WH, Lawson DL, Saldeen TGP. 1989. Impaired coronary vasodilator response to acetylcholine and bradykinin after occlusion-reperfusion. Circ Res 64:43–54.
5. Furchtgott RF, Zawadski J. 1980. The obligatory role of endothelial cells on the relaxation of arterial smooth muscle by acetylcholine. Nature (Lond) 288:373–376.
6. Furchtgott RF, Vanhoutte PM. 1989. Endothelium-derived relaxing and contracting factors. FASEB J 3:2007–2018.
7. Mehta JL, Lawson DL, Nichols WW. 1989. Attenuated coronary relaxation after reperfusion: Effects of superoxide dismutase and TxA_2 inhibitor U-63557. Am J Physiol 257: H1240–H1246.
8. Kloner RA, Ganote CE, Jennings RB. 1974. The "no-reflow" phenomenon after temporary coronary occlusion in the dog. J Clin Invest 54:1496–1508.
9. Ambrosio G, Weisman HF, Mannisi IA, Becker LC. 1989. Progressive impairment of regional myocardial perfusion after initial restoration of postischemic blood flow. Circulation 80:1846–1861.
10. Przyklenk K, Kloner RA. 1989. "Reperfusion injury" by oxygen-derived free radicals? Effect of superoxidase dismutase + catalase, given at the time of reperfusion on myocardial infarct size, contractile function, coronary microvasculature and regional myocardial blood flow. Circ Res 64:86–96.
11. Engler RL, Schmid-Schonbein GW, Pavlec RS. 1983. Leukocyte capillary plugging in myocardial ischemia and reperfusion in the dog. Am J Pathol 111:98–111.
12. Kloner RA, Alker KJ. 1984. The effect of streptokinase on the intramyocardial hemorrhage, infarct size and the no-reflow phenomenon during reperfusion. Circulation 70: 513–521.
13. Kloner RA, Rude RE, Carlson N, Maroko PR, DeBoer LWV, Braunwald E. 1980. Ultrastructural evidence of microvascular damage and myocardial cell injury after coronary artery occlusion. Which comes first? Circulation 62:945–952.
14. Heyndrickx GR, Baig H, Nellens P, Lensen I, Fishbein MC, Vatner SF. 1978. Depression of regional blood flow and wall thickening after brief coronary occlusions. Am J Physiol 234:H653–H659.
15. Vanhaecke J, Flameng W, Borgers M, Jang IK, Van de Wert F, DeGeest H. 1990. Evidence for decreased coronary flow reserve in viable postischemic myocardium. Circ Res 67: 1201–1210.

16. Liu GS, Thornton J, Van Winkle DM, Stanley AWH, Olsson RA, Downey JM. 1991. Protection against infarction afforded by preconditioning is mediated by A_1 adenosine receptors in rabbit heart. Circulation 84:350–356.
17. Thornton JD, Liu GS, Olsson RA, Downey JM. 1992. Intravenous pretreatment with A_1-selective adenosine analogues protects the heart against infarction. Circulation 85:659–665.
18. Berne RM. 1980. The role of adenosine in the regulation of coronary flow. Circ Res 47:807–813.
19. Olafsson B, Forman MB, Puett DW, Pon A, Cates CHU, Friesinger GC, Virmani R. 1987. Reduction of reperfusion injury in the canine preparation by intraoronary adenosine: Importance of the endothelium and the no-reflow phenomenon. Circulation 5:1135–1145.
20. Bauer B, Simkhovich B, Kloner RA, Przyklenk K. 1993. Does preconditioning protect the coronary vasculature from subsequent ischemia/reperfusion injury? Circulation 88:659–672.
21. Nichols WW, Mehta JL, Donnelly WH, Lawson D, Thompson L, ter Riet M. 1989. Reduction in coronary vasodilator reserve following coronary occlusion and reperfusion in anesthetized dogs: Role of endothelium-derived relaxing factor, myocardial neutrophil infiltration and prostaglandins. J Mol Cell Cardiol 20:943–954.
22. DeFily DV, Chilian WM. 1991. Preconditioning protects coronary microvascular endothelial function. Circulation 84(Suppl II):II434 (abstr).
23. DeFily DV, Chilian WM. 1993. Preconditioning protects coronary arteriolar endothelium from ischemia-reperfusion injury. Am J Physiol 265:H700–H706.
24. Stahl LD, Aversano TR, Becker LC. 1986. Selective enhancement of function of stunned myocardium by increased flow. Circulation 74:843–851.
25. Laxson DD, Homans DC, Dai XZ, Sublett E, Bache RJ. 1989. Oxygen consumption and coronary reactivity in postischemic myocardium. Circ Res 64:9–20.
26. Schott RJ, Rohmann S, Braun ER, Shaper W. 1990. Ischemic preconditioning reduces infarct size in swine myocardium. Circ Res 66:1133–1142.
27. Ovize M, Kloner RA, Hale SL, Przyklenk K. 1992. Coronary cyclic flow variations "precondition" ischemic myocardium. Circulation 85:779–789.
28. Gross GJ, Auchampach JA. 1992. Blockade of ATP-sensitive potassium channels prevents myocardial preconditioning in dogs. Circ Res 70:223–233.
29. Hale SL, Kloner RA. 1992. Effect of ischemic preconditioning on regional myocardial flow in the rabbit heart. Coronary Artery Dis 3:133–140.
30. Downey J, Liu Guang. 1992. Acetylcholine preconditions rabbit heart: Further evidence for G_i protein coupling in preconditioning. Circulation 86(Suppl I):I174 (abstr).
31. Kitakaze M, Hori M, Takashima S, Sato H, Inoue M, Kamada T. 1993. Ischemic preconditioning increases adenosine release and 5′-nucleotidase activity during myocardial ischemia and reperfusion in dogs: Implications for myocardial salvage. Circulation 87:208–215.

II. MECHANISMS OF CARDIOPROTECTION BY PRECONDITIONING: THEORIES AND CONTROVERSIES

5. ROLE OF ALTERED ENERGY METABOLISM IN ISCHEMIC PRECONDITIONING

KEITH A. REIMER, RICHARD S. VANDER HEIDE,
CHARLES E. MURRY, and ROBERT B. JENNINGS

INTRODUCTION: ISCHEMIC PRECONDITIONING AS AN ADAPTATION TO STRESS

Myocardium that is exposed to a mild, sublethal stress is capable of undergoing adaptive changes that enable it to better tolerate a more severe, potentially lethal exposure to the same (or different) form of stress. This response may be rapid (minutes) or delayed (hours). For example, when animals are exposed to heat stress, the myocardium responds by synthesizing a family of heat shock proteins (HSPs) [1,2], which, 24 hours later, are associated with an increased tolerance to various insults, including heat stress and ischemia [3–6] (see Chapter 6).

In 1986 we reported [7] that myocardium exposed to a series of four 5-minute episodes of ischemia, each separated by 5 minutes of reperfusion, responded differently to a sustained episode of ischemia than did virgin myocardium. A rapid adaptation to ischemia had occurred, such that when this preconditioned myocardium was exposed 5 minutes later to a sustained, 40-minute period of ischemia and then reperfused, the extent of necrosis was only 25% of the expected infarct size. We termed this phenomenon *ischemic preconditioning*. This phenomenon now has been reproduced in several animal species, including dogs [7,8], pigs [9], rabbits [10–12], and rats [13–15]. The general biology of preconditioning's effect on myocardial infarct size is reviewed in detail in Chapter 1 of this book.

The increased resistance to lethal cell injury is accompanied by a reduced rate of ischemic metabolism. In particular, both the depletion of adenosine triphosphate (ATP) stores and the accumulation of products of anaerobic glycolysis occur more slowly during the early phase of the sustained test episode [16]. Thus, in this chapter we shall concentrate on the metabolic features of preconditioning, because it seems likely that an understanding of the metabolic changes associated with this phenomenon will lead to an understanding of the pathogenesis of the preconditioned state.

ENERGY RELEASE AND UTILIZATION IN ISCHEMIC MYOCARDIUM

Our analysis of the metabolic changes in ischemia will be restricted to those changes seen in severe or total ischemia. The major pathways through which ATP is produced and utilized in severely or totally ischemic myocardium are summarized in Figure 1.

Energy supply

Under aerobic conditions, virtually all myocardial high energy phosphate (HEP) is produced by oxidative phosphorylation (Figure 1). However, oxi-

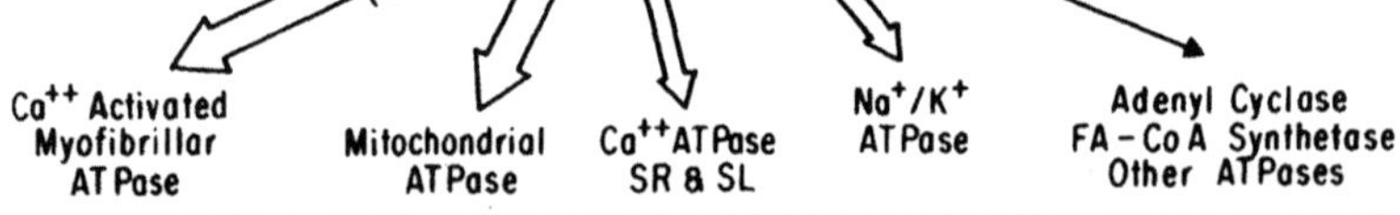

Figure 1. The principal reactions producing and utilizing high energy phosphates in ischemic myocardium. The width of the arrows indicates the estimated quantitative importance of the various reactions. In severe ischemia, aerobic respiration is abolished. The preexisting stores of high energy phosphate, in the form of creatine phosphate (CP) and adenosine triphosphate (ATP), are relatively small. Thus, anaerobic glycolysis becomes the principal source of energy, producing about 80% of the high-energy phosphate bonds that can be utilized by severely ischemic tissue (see Table 1). Substrate level phosphorylation of alpha-ketoglutarate in the mitochondria does not require oxygen, but the tissue content of substrates that can be shuttled to alpha-ketoglutarate is small. Energy utilization also is reduced markedly during ischemia. Cardiac contraction consumes much of the ATP produced in aerobic myocardium. The energy used for contractile effort includes the Ca^{++}-activated myofibrillar ATPase reaction as well as reactions involving cycling of calcium across the sarcoplasmic reticulum and sarcolemma. However, contraction is depressed markedly in areas of severe ischemia. ATP is required for transport ATPases such as the Na/K ATPase and calcium ATPases responding to the continuous electrical stimulation of the left ventricle and for a variety of other cellular processes. Finally, recent studies have shown that a major source of ATP utilization during ischemia is the squandering of ATP by the mitochondrial ATPase (reverse function of the ATP synthetase). Modified from a figure in Jennings and Reimer [104].

Table 1. Potential sources of high energy phosphate (HEP) in myocardium at the onset of total ischemia

	HEP production (μmol/g dry wt)
Metabolizable substrate	
Glucose from glycogen	612
(204 μmol G × 3 μmol HEP/μmol G)	
Glucose of extracellular H_2O	7
(3.5 μmol G × 2 μmol HEP/μmol G)	
Mitochondrial substrate level phosphorylation	5
(Glutamate, α-ketoglutarate, etc.)	
Total	624
Reserves of HEP	
ATP	52
(26 μmol × 2 μmol HEP/μmol ATP)	
ADP	3
(3 μmol × 1 μmol HEP/μmol ADP)	
CP	40
(40 μmol × 1 μmol HEP/μmol CP)	
Other	2
(GTP, CTP, and UTP, etc.)	
Total	97

The total HEP available from all sources to totally ischemic myocardium is estimated from known levels of myocardial substrate and HEP reserves. The principal source of new HEP is anaerobic glycolysis, using glucose from the 204 ± 10 μmoles glucosyl equivalents of glycogen in control left ventricle. An extracellular glucose of 3.5 μmol/g dry weight is based on a serum glucose of 5.5 mM.
G, glucose; ATP, adenosine triphosphate; ADP, adenosine diphosphate; CP, creatine phosphate; GTP, guanosine triphosphate; CTP, cytidine triphosphate; UTP, uridine triphosphate.
Reprinted with permission from Jennings et al. [103].

dative phosphorylation ceases when the O_2 supply becomes exhausted, some 8–10 seconds after the onset of severe ischemia. The myocardium then utilizes the reserve HEP found in creatine phosphate (CP), ATP, adenosine diphosphate (ADP), and the small residual amounts of guanine, cytidine and uridine nucleotides.

The major energy reserves of myocardium are stored in the form of glycogen. In dogs, cardiac glycogen ranges from 130 to 300 μmol glucose equivalents/g dry weight. In addition, a small amount of glucose (about 1.7–3.5 μmol/g dry weight) is trapped in the extracellular space at the onset of ischemia. Small quantities of mitochondrial substrates also exist that may be phosphorylated through shuttle mechanisms.

The total HEP potentially available from all sources to totally ischemic myocardium is presented in Table 1. We estimate that about 100 μmol/g dry weight of HEP are present at the onset of ischemia and that an additional 600 μmol can be produced by way of energy release from stored substrates, primarily from anaerobic glycolysis using glucose-1-phosphate from glycogen.

Energy demand

Under aerobic conditions, most of the HEP is consumed supporting the contractile process (Figure 1). When effective contraction ceases 8–10 seconds after the onset of ischemia, some energy probably is utilized in the attempt of the myocytes to contract in response to continuing electrical activation. In addition, whether or not effective contraction occurs, these electrical stimuli cause Na^+, K^+, and Ca^{2+} ion cycling, which drives the various ion transport ATPases [17]. These energy-consuming reactions are reactions that occur under aerobic conditions and continue at reduced rates under ischemic conditions. However, a major route of ATP consumption in ischemia is a reaction that does not occur in aerobic myocardium, namely, mitochondrial ATPase activity.

The mitochondrial ATPase is identical to the mitochondrial ATP synthetase, which is present as a macromolecular complex (F1-F0 particles) in the cristae of the mitochondria [18]. When mitochondria are energized during aerobic metabolism, this enzyme complex synthesizes ATP from adenosine diphosphate (ADP) and inorganic phosphate (Pi). However, when the mitochondria are deenergized under the conditions of myocardial ischemia, the synthetase reaction reverses and ATP is hydrolyzed to ADP and Pi. The contribution of the mitochondrial ATPase to energy utilization in ischemia has been studied only recently [19,20]. When compared to nontreated ischemic tissue from the same heart, totally ischemic myocardium pretreated with oligomycin, a potent inhibitor of the ATPase, maintained a higher net ATP throughout the first 90 minutes of ischemia [20]; in fact, the rate of ATP depletion was reduced by up to 50%. Thus, this reaction is a previously unrecognized major factor in the supply–demand relationship of ischemic myocardium. Moreover, ATP depletion would occur even more quickly during ischemia, were it not for a small molecular weight protein inhibitor present in mitochondria of "slow heart rate" species, including dogs, the so-called F1-ATPase inhibitory subunit (IF1) [21]. When tissue becomes acidotic during ischemia, this inhibitor binds to the mitochondrial ATPase and slows the rate of ATP degradation.

Supply–demand imbalance in ischemia

An important feature of severe or total ischemia is that there appears to be tight coupling between the rate of anaerobic glycolysis and the rate of HEP utilization. The nature of this coupling is such that the supply of HEP always is inadequate to meet the demand. During the initial few minutes of ischemia, both ATP utilization and anaerobic glycolysis proceed relatively rapidly. However, after 10–15 minutes of ischemia, the rates of ATP utilization, anaerobic glycolysis, and net HEP depletion all are reduced. Although it has long been known that anaerobic glycolysis may be inhibited by the decreasing pH and accumulating products of this pathway [22,23], the ex-

Table 2. High energy phosphate (HEP) utilization in low-flow ischemia

Ischemic interval (min after onset)	HEP utilization (μmol/g/dry wt/min)
0–1.5	68.5
1.5–5	24.3
5–10	12.6
10–15	14.9
15–20	11.4
20–40	4.2

HEP utilization was calculated from measurements of CP, ATP, ADP, and lactate at the beginning and end of each time interval, assuming that utilization is the sum of HEP depletion from existing reserves plus HEP production through anaerobic glycolysis, as estimated by changes in tissue lactate content (all measured in μmol/g/dry weight). Thus HEP utilization was calculated at the interval change in the following equation: [2 × (26 − observed ATP)] + [3 − observed ADP] + [40 − observed CP] + 1.5 × (observed lactate − 8)]. (Abbreviations as in Table 1.) The measurements were made in samples of severely ischemic (≤0.07 ml/min/g wet wt) subendocardial myocardium obtained following occlusion of the circumflex coronary artery of dogs in vivo. Reproduced with permission from Jennings et al. [103].

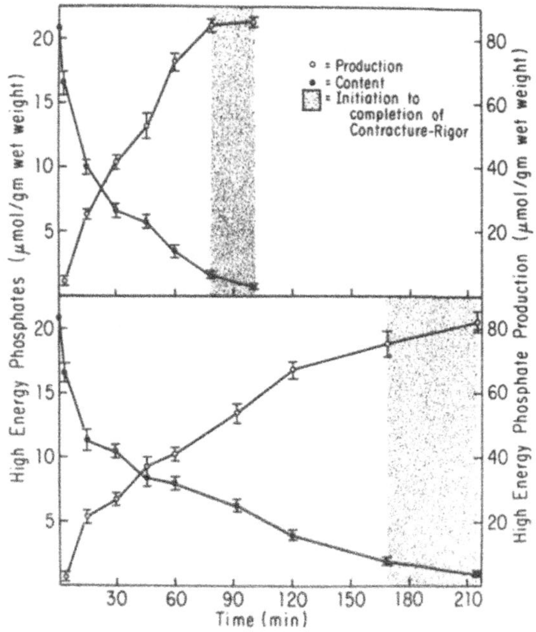

Figure 2. Effect of temperature on myocardial high-energy phosphate production and depletion during total ischemia, in vitro, at 37°C (top panel) and 28°C (bottom panel). The cumulative high energy phosphate (HEP) production via anaerobic glycolysis was calculated from the changing tissue content of lactate (HEP = 1.5 × observed change in lactate). The reserve myocardial HEP content was calculated as (observed CP + [2 × observed ATP] + ADP). ATP = adenosine triphosphate; ADP = adenosine diphosphate. Brackets indicate the standard errors of the mean. Reprinted with permission from Jones et al. [24].

planation for the coupling between the decreasing rate of HEP utilization (Table 2) and the decreasing rate of anaerobic glycolysis during ischemia remains unknown. Moreover, all interventions that slow ATP utilization, such as hypothermia [24] and oligomycin [20], also slow energy release via anaerobic glycolysis (as measured by the rate of tissue lactate accumulation; Figure 2). Thus it has not been possible to prevent ATP depletion because it has not been possible to slow ATP depletion without also slowing anaerobic glycolysis.

METABOLIC AND GENERAL BIOLOGIC FEATURES OF ISCHEMIC PRECONDITIONING

Altered energy metabolism in preconditioned myocardium

The effect of ischemic preconditioning on myocardial metabolite levels is similar regardless of the specific protocol used to achieve preconditioning. In each case, the myocardium resumes aerobic metabolism and the adenylate charge quickly is restored to a normal value of 0.9 [25]. The nucleosides, bases, lactate, and glycolytic intermediates that have accumulated during the preconditioning episode of ischemia are either reutilized or washed to the systemic circulation and their myocardial concentration is restored to control (Table 3). The total adenine nucleotide pool is reduced in direct relation to the duration of preceding ischemia; the longer the ischemia, the lower the pool.

Table 3. Constituents and catabolites of the adenine nucleotide pool following 5 minutes of ischemia or ischemic preconditioning

	Control	5I	5I + 20R	(5I + 5R) × 4
ATP	25.87 ± 0.42	13.30 ± 1.46	19.61 ± 1.29	18.13 ± 0.96
ADP	4.33 ± 0.34	8.36 ± 0.60	4.14 ± 0.58	2.59 ± 0.21
AMP	0.50 ± 0.07	3.28 ± 0.63	0.66 ± 0.17	0.31 ± 0.04
Total AN	30.41 ± 0.38	24.94 ± 1.36	24.41 ± 1.28	21.02 ± 1.08
Adenosine	0.007 ± 0.006	1.191 ± 0.390	0.00	0.00
Inosine	0.019 ± 0.012	5.704 ± 1.995	0.092 ± 0.086	0.00
Hypoxanthine	0.026 ± 0.024	0.684 ± 0.170	0.096 ± 0.090	0.009 ± 0.009
Xanthine	0.026 ± 0.024	0.446 ± 0.082	0.035 ± 0.022	0.071 ± 0.016
Total AN + NS	30.46 ± 0.40	32.97 ± 2.04	24.52 ± 1.19	21.10 ± 1.07
n	12	5	5	5

Metabolites were measured in the subendocardial zone of canine left ventricular myocardium of nonischemic (control) and ischemic or preconditioned regions. The ischemic or preconditioned samples were each from areas with collateral blood flow ≤0.10 ml/min/g. Ischemic preconditioning was achieved either by one 5-minute period of ischemia, followed by 20 minutes of reperfusion (5I + 20R) or by four cycles of 5 minutes of ischemia followed by 5 minutes of reperfusion. The data were obtained as part of the studies reported in references [16,60].

AN, adenine nucleotides; NS, adenine nucleosides; I, ischemia; R, reperfusion; other abbreviations as in Table 1.

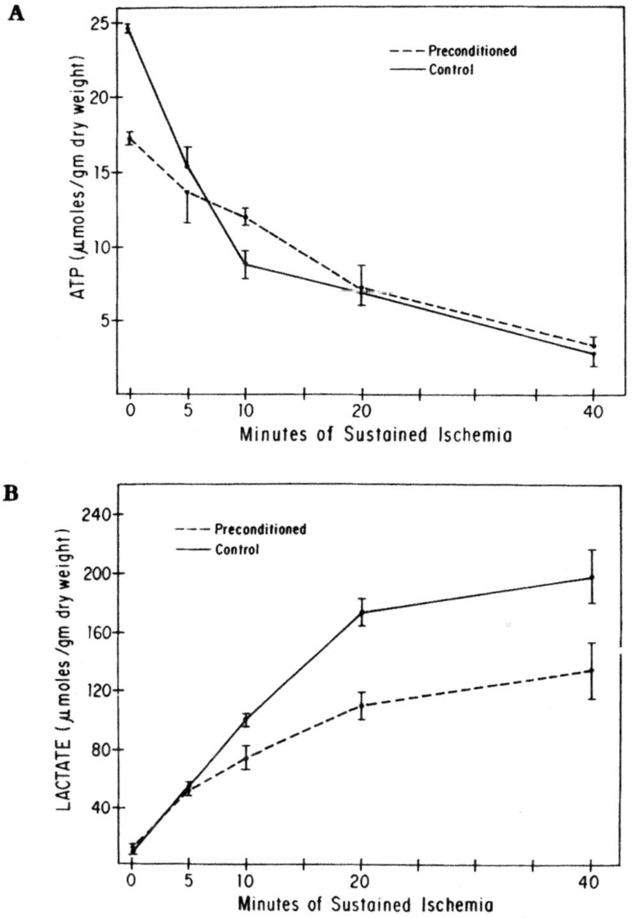

Figure 3. Subendocardial adenosine triphosphate (ATP) content (**A**) or subendocardial lactate content (**B**) vs. duration of ischemia in control and ischemically preconditioned myocardium. In control myocardium, ATP depletion was most rapid during the initial 10 minutes of ischemia and slowed thereafter. Preconditioned myocardium had less ATP than control at the onset of the sustained occlusion. However, because the subsequent rate of ATP depletion was substantially slower, by 10 minutes, ATP content was significantly higher in preconditioned myocardium vs. controls ($p < 0.01$). Concomitantly, the rate of lactate accumulation was substantially slower in preconditioned vs. control myocardium. The data was obtained from groups with similarly severe ischemia, including only dogs with subendocardial flow ≤0.07 ml/min · g. Reprinted with permission from Murry et al. [16].

There are three other notable metabolic differences between preconditioned and control myocardium. First, creatine phosphate content in preconditioned myocardium substantially exceeds control (the creatine phosphate overshoot). For example, after 12 minutes of ischemia and 10 minutes of reperfusion, creatine phosphate is 35% greater than control [26]. This cre-

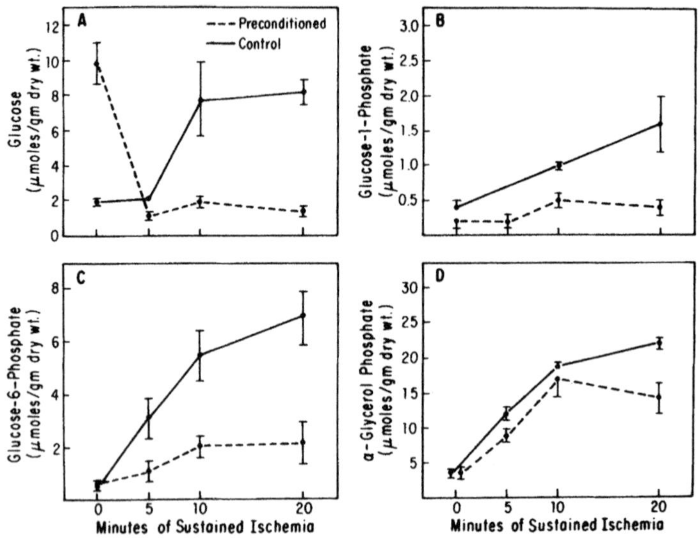

Figure 4. Glycolytic metabolite content in control and ischemically preconditioned myocardium. The data were obtained from subendocardial samples, all of which had collateral blood flow ≤0.10 ml/min/g. **A**: Glucose (G). In control myocardium, G increased steadily during the first 20 minutes of ischemia, probably as a result of debrancher enzyme activity liberating glucose rather than glucose-1-phosphate (G-1-P) from the glucose-1,6 linkages found in glycogen branch points. This intracellular G is metabolized slowly when sarcoplasmic ATP is low. In preconditioned myocardium, G content was increased significantly at the onset of ischemia. Most of this increase is probably attributable to the glucose remaining from glycogenolysis occurring during the preconditioning episode of ischemia. Much of this excess glucose in preconditioned myocardium disappeared after 5 minutes of ischemia. **B**: G-1-P. **C**: Glucose-6-phosphate. **D**: Alpha-glycerol phosphate. Note that accumulation of G-1-P, G-6-P, and alpha-glycerol phosphate each increased more slowly in preconditioned than control ischemic myocardium. In conjunction with the slower accumulation of lactate (Figure 3B), these results reflect a slower rate of anaerobic glycolysis in preconditioned myocardium. Reprinted with permission from Murry et al. [16].

atine phosphate overshoot persists for at least 1 hour, but it has not been determined when it disappears. Second, tissue glucose is four times greater than control (Figure 4) [16]. Most of this excess glucose is thought to be intracellular, although some may be associated with an increased plasma or interstitial fluid volume. Third, the tissue is edematous [16,27] and has a higher content of potassium than control tissue. The tissue edema is thought to be intracellular because it persists well after the phase of reactive hyperemia [16,28].

The effect of ischemic preconditioning on the energy supply–demand relationship during a subsequent episode of ischemia has been studied in severe ischemia in vivo [16] and total ischemia in vitro [29]. The results in vivo with respect to ATP and lactate are shown in Figure 3. Much less ATP was utilized in the preconditioned myocardium during the first 10 minutes of ischemia than was utilized in the virgin control heart (Figure 3A). The accumulation of lactate (Figure 3B), and all glycolytic metabolites except alpha glycerophosphate, also was significantly depressed (Figure 4). Thus, preconditioning eliminates the high initial rate of myocardial energy metabolism seen in ischemic control myocardium. Consideration of the major pathways through which ATP is produced and utilized in ischemic myocardium (Figure 1) indicates that the slowed depletion of ATP during ischemia in preconditioned myocardium hypothetically could be due either to increased production of HEP or to slowed energy utilization. However, increased production of HEP does not seem tenable for the reasons discussed in the following paragraphs.

First, production of high energy phosphates could be increased if preconditioning opened preexisting collateral channels so that more collateral flow, and thus more oxygen, could reach the ischemic tissue. When anaerobic glycolysis is used to produce ATP from glycogen, only 3 µmoles of ATP are generated for each µmole of glucose-1-phosphate converted to lactate. This contrasts with 38 µmoles of ATP that can be produced if the same glucosyl unit is oxidized completely to CO_2 and H_2O [30]. Thus, a relatively small increment in collateral blood flow could have substantial benefit for energy production. In addition, improved collateral flow could facilitate anaerobic glycolysis by washing out the catabolites, which cause feedback inhibition of this pathway.

Although it has been shown that repetitive brief coronary occlusions, conducted over a course of days, induces growth of collaterals [31], when only one to four brief occlusions comprise the preconditioning protocol an immediate increase in collateral blood flow would not be expected and has not been observed [7]. Moreover, the marked limitation of infarct size achieved with preconditioning has been observed when control and preconditioned hearts are matched for the same collateral blood flow during the test episode of ischemia [7,32]. In addition, the fact that preconditioning has been observed in pigs, rabbits, and rats — species with minimal native collateral blood flow — also argues against a collateral flow-mediated mechanism. Finally, the metabolic slowing observed in vivo also has been observed in myocardium that was preconditioned in vivo and subsequently subjected to total (no-flow) ischemia in vitro [29].

Second, high energy phosphate depletion might be delayed if cellular stores of high energy phosphates were higher at the onset of the test episode of ischemia. It is known that a transient episode (e.g., 10–15 minutes) of ischemia, followed by reperfusion, results in an overshoot in creatine phosphate content by up to 170% of baseline [28,33]. On the other hand, this increase in creatine phosphate is counterbalanced by a partial depletion of ATP and ADP [20,25,28]; thus the net high energy phosphate content of preconditioned myocardium at the onset of the test episode of ischemia is no greater than control [16,20].

Third, ATP production could be increased during ischemia if the rate of anaerobic glycolysis were increased. In support of this hypothesis, adenosine, a proposed mediator of ischemic preconditioning (see below), has been shown to accelerate glycolytic flux in isolated perfused rat hearts [34]. However, this effect of adenosine is unlikely to occur in in vivo models of severe ischemia where the rate of anaerobic glycolysis is quickly slowed by tissue acidosis and other accumulating metabolites of the glycolytic pathway [22,35]. In addition, as reviewed above, *slowing*, rather than stimulation of anaerobic glycolysis, during the test episode of ischemia is one of the hallmarks of preconditioned myocardium in dogs [16]. A similar slowing of anaerobic glycolysis has been reported in preconditioned ischemic rat hearts, and the slowing has been proposed to be a consequence of partial depletion of glycogen during preconditioning [36]. These studies also showed that repletion of glycogen subsequent to preconditioning occurred in parallel with the time course of the loss of myocardial protection.

Reports from studies of isolated perfused rodent hearts have concluded that preconditioning improved postischemic recovery of function when the reperfusate included the glycolytic substrate glucose, but not when postischemic metabolism was supported only by a mitochondrial substrate, pyruvate [37,38]. Whether such substrate effects during reperfusion pertain in any way to the effects of ischemic preconditioning on infarct size in intact animal models is uncertain, but it is obvious that events during reperfusion in vivo cannot explain the effect of preconditioning on metabolism during the preceding period of ischemia. Moreover, another preliminary report has *not* confirmed that reperfusion of rabbit hearts with a buffer containing pyruvate rather than glucose had any effect on the infarct-limiting effect of ischemic preconditioning [39].

From these considerations, it is quite unlikely that the energy-sparing effects of ischemic preconditioning are explained by increased high-energy phosphate production during the test episode of ischemia. On the contrary, the slower rate of high-energy phosphate depletion during ischemia is likely explained by a slowing of one or more energy utilizing reactions. Thus, exposure of myocardium to a brief stress (ischemia) results in a rapid adaptation, which is characterized by a decreased energy utilization by one or multiple metabolic pathways during a subsequent episode of ischemia. The effect is a reduction in the demand of the ischemic tissue for HEP which results in slowed depletion of HEP, slowed accumulation of lactate (the principal component of the osmotic load), and delayed development of lethal ischemic injury.

If so, it follows that a proposed mechanism to explain the protection against necrosis must also explain the metabolic effects of preconditioning. Consequently, much of the remainder of this chapter will focus on proposed mechanisms of preconditioning from this point of view. There are two facets of the preconditioning phenomenon that need to be considered: (1) What subcellular pathways are altered to slow ischemic energy metabolism in myocardium that has been preconditioned? and (2) what is the signal produced by ischemia through which this reduced energy demand is achieved?

General biology of ischemic preconditioning

Consideration of the possible answers to the two preceding questions regarding the characteristic alterations in energy demand in preconditioned myocardium may be simplified to some degree by the knowledge that the mechanism of preconditioning also must be consistent with the general biology of the phenomenon (see Chapter 1). Briefly, the biology of preconditioning in dogs can be summarized as follows: (1) Preconditioning can be achieved with only one preliminary episode of ischemia, which need not exceed 5 minutes [8] and may be achieved with as little as 90 seconds of ischemia (R.S. Vander Heide and K.A. Reimer, unreported observations). (2) By definition, at least momentary reperfusion between the preconditioning episode and test episode is required; otherwise the preconditioning period would simply prolong the duration of the test episode of ischemia. The minimum duration of reperfusion is certainly no more than 5 minutes and evidence from the dog (K.A. Reimer et al., unreported observations) and rat [40] models indicates that this necessary period of reflow may be as short as 30–60 seconds. (3) The adaptive change is relatively short-lived, in that if the time of reperfusion between preconditioning and the test episode of ischemia is extended to 2 or more hours, the protective effect dissipates [32]. (4) Preconditioning *delays*, but does not *prevent*, lethal cell injury; i.e., infarct size is limited if measured after a test episode of 40–60 minutes, but if the test episode is extended to 90 or more minutes, the protective effect of preconditioning dissipates [7,41]. These general considerations also apply in species other than the dog, although the specific time limits may vary slightly.

WHAT ENERGY-CONSUMING PATHWAYS ARE SLOWED IN PRECONDITIONED MYOCARDIUM?

Many cellular processes and reactions contribute to the progressive decline in ATP during ischemia. Those thought to be of particular importance are shown in the bottom half of Figure 1 and include continued attempts at contraction, transport ATPases, continued cycling of the fatty acid CoA synthetase, adenylate cyclase, and the mitochondrial ATPase (reverse function of the mitochondrial ATP synthase). However, at present the relative contribution of each of these various processes to overall ATP utilization is not clear, nor is it known which of these, if any, might be slowed in preconditioned myocardium.

Inhibition of mitochondrial ATPase

It is hypothetically possible that inhibition of the mitochondrial ATPase might play a role in the reduced demand for high-energy phosphate induced

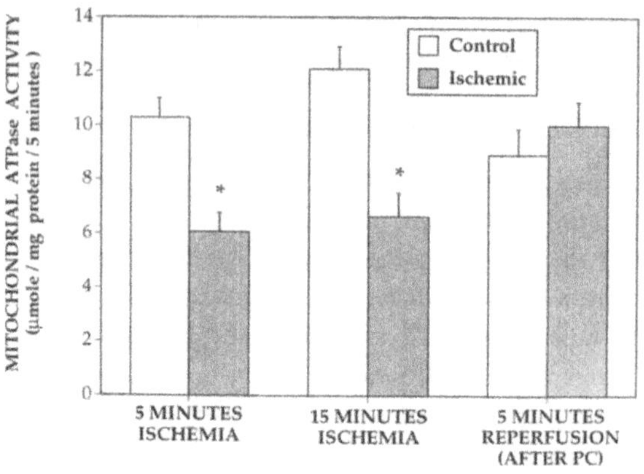

Figure 5. Effect of ischemia and ischemia plus reperfusion on mitochondrial ATPase activity. Ischemia was induced by circumflex coronary occlusion in anesthetized open-chest dogs. The heart then was excised and submitochondrial particles were prepared from subendocardial samples of ischemic and nonischemic control regions. After 5 minutes of ischemia, mitochondrial ATPase activity was reduced by about 50%, and was not further affected by prolonging the ischemic period to 15 minutes. However, mitochondrial ATPase activity was restored to control by 5 minutes of reperfusion after preconditioning with four 5-minute episodes of ischemia. Thus, early inhibition of the mitochondrial ATPase in ischemia is an endogenous cardioprotectant mechanism, which occurs even in nonpreconditioned myocardium. However, the fact that this inhibition does not persist during reperfusion indicates that the energy-sparing effect of ischemic preconditioning cannot be explained by inhibition of the mitochondrial ATPase at the onset of the test episode of ischemia. From data reported in Vander Heide et al. [42].

by ischemic preconditioning. This might occur if either (1) ischemic preconditioning somehow alters the ATPase-inhibitor binding site such that during the test episode of ischemia the inhibitor would bind more quickly or completely than it does in nonpreconditioned ischemic myocardium, or (2) some or all of the inhibitor that bound to the ATPase during the preconditioning episode of ischemia remained bound during the phase of arterial reperfusion.

However, we observed in a recent study of the role of the ATPase in ischemia [42] that (1) mitochondrial ATPase activity is significantly inhibited very quickly (within 90 seconds) following the onset of severe ischemia in vivo, (2) the ATPase activity is inhibited to its full extent by only 5 minutes of ischemia, and (3) inhibition does not persist following arterial reperfusion (Figure 5). The lack of persistent inhibition during reperfusion also has been observed by other investigators [43,44]. Thus, inhibition of the mitochondrial ATPase cannot be used to explain the energy-sparing effects of ischemic preconditioning.

Additional support for the conclusion that inhibition of the mitochondrial ATPase does *not* explain the energy-sparing effect of ischemic preconditioning comes from observations that ischemic preconditioning against lethal cell injury occurs in rat myocardium in vivo [13,14]. It is known that myocardium of rodents with fast heart rates (i.e., rats, mice, and hamsters) contains only 20–30% as much of the endogenous inhibitor (IF1) as mammals with slower heart rates (rabbits, dogs, pigs, and humans) [45]. Thus, in rats mitochondrial ATP hydrolysis is slowed very little at the start of ischemia. That rat myocardium can be preconditioned despite markedly reduced mitochondrial ATPase inhibitor activity [13,15] is further evidence against the hypothesis that altered mitochondrial ATPase activity explains the metabolic slowing induced by ischemic preconditioning.

Concomitant myocardial stunning

In aerobic myocardium, most of the ATP produced is utilized by metabolic reactions involved in contractile function. Shortly after the onset of ischemia, contractile function is depressed markedly, although in isolated heats subjected to global ischemia feeble attempts to contract can be detected for several minutes [17]. Furthermore, electrical activation continues to elicit some calcium cycling, which contributes to ATP utilization during ischemia. The one or more brief episodes of ischemia that induces the preconditioning effect also causes myocardial stunning. (*Stunning* refers to the reduced systolic contractile function that develops in reperfused myocardium that has been subjected to a brief episode of ischemia, even though the ischemic injury is insufficient to cause myocardial necrosis [46,47].) Thus, we postulated that, because of concomitant stunning, preconditioned myocardium might have reduced contractile effort, and therefore less energy expenditure in the initial phase of the test episode of ischemia. Indirect evidence supporting this hypothesis comes from the observation that a brief episode of ischemia resulted in a more rapid onset of contractile failure during a subsequent episode [48].

Is the presence of myocardial stunning sufficient to achieve the protective effect of preconditioning?

Studies using either dogs, pigs, or rabbits [32,49,50] have shown that the cardioprotective effect of preconditioning is a relatively transient phenomenon that dissipates after an hour or two. Stunning, however, may persist for many hours. For example, we have observed that when the reperfusion period between preconditioning and test episodes of ischemia was extended to 2 hours, cellular protection was partially lost even though severe stunning still was present [32]. These results indicate that the presence of stunning alone is *insufficient* to achieve the full protective effect of ischemic preconditioning. However, they do not eliminate the possibility that stunning may be a *necessary* prerequisite for cardiac protection.

Is stunning necessary to achieve preconditioning?

Four 5-minute episodes of coronary occlusion, which formed the first preconditioning protocol, cause relatively mild stunning [51]. The discrepancy between the mild degree of stunning and the marked limitation of infarct size is indirect evidence that preconditioning is not simply a consequence of stunning. Other studies have provided direct evidence that stunning is not necessary for preconditioning to occur. For example, we tested the effects of preconditioning in vivo on myocardial metabolism during a subsequent period of total ischemia in vitro [52]. After preconditioning in vivo, hearts were arrested with KCl to abolish all electrical and contractile activity and then were extirpated and subjected to total ischemia in vitro. The initial rates of both ATP depletion and anaerobic glycolysis were much slower in preconditioned than in control myocardium from the same hearts. Thus, the difference in ischemic metabolism between control and preconditioned tissue persisted despite abolition of possible differences in contractile effort during early ischemia.

Further evidence against a causal relation between stunning and precon-

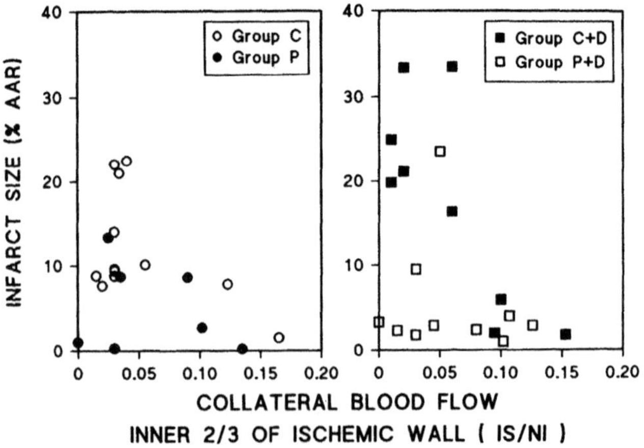

Figure 6. Effect of restoring contractile function before the test episode of ischemia on the infarct-limiting effect of preconditioning. Infarct size is plotted vs. collateral blood flow, normalized to simultaneously measured nonischemic flow (ischemic/nonischemic; IS/NI). In group C (nonpreconditioned control hearts), there was an inverse relation between infarct size and collateral blood flow. Infarct size was smaller in group P (preconditioned hearts) vs. C, using analysis of covariance with collateral blood flow as an independent variable and infarct size as a dependent variable ($p < 0.05$). Infarct size was not different (p = N.S.) between group P+D (preconditioned hearts in which regional contractile function was restored using dobutamine) and group P using either flow parameter. Infarct size in group C+D (nonpreconditioned control hearts treated with dobutamine) was larger than in group C when absolute collateral blood flow was used in the analysis of covariance (data not shown), but this difference was abolished when normalized flow data were used. Thus, restoration of contractile function in preconditioned myocardium prior to the test episode of ischemia did not abolish the cardioprotective effect of preconditioning. Reprinted with permission from Matsuda et al. [51].

ditioning is provided by a recent study in our laboratory [51]. In this study, dobutamine was administered after our standard preconditioning protocol to overcome the postischemic contractile dysfunction (stunning) associated with preconditioning. Although dobutamine infusion easily restored contractile function to baseline values, the protective effect of ischemic preconditioning on infarct size was preserved (Figure 6). Thus, reduced contractile effort, per se, at the onset of the test episode of ischemia was not required for ischemic preconditioning. However, this study was not designed to *prevent* stunning from occurring. Since dobutamine was not administered until after the preconditioning protocol, it most likely did not correct the underlying cellular defect that caused the contractile dysfunction. Thus, these results do not exclude the possibility that an underlying cellular defect that causes the contractile dysfunction of stunning could also cause the cardioprotective effect of preconditioning; i.e., that stunning and ischemic preconditioning might be caused by a common underlying mechanism. However, in pigs preconditioned with two 10-minute episodes of ischemia, pretreatment with nifedipine prevented myocardial stunning but did not cause larger infarcts [53]. Similarly, it has been reported that ischemic preconditioning can be achieved in rabbits [50] or dogs [54] using brief episodes of ischemia that do not cause significant stunning (see Chapter 3).

Adenosine

A growing body of evidence suggests that adenosine produced during preconditioning episodes of ischemia may serve as the signal to reduce the activity of one or more pathways contributing to myocardial energy demand during subsequent periods of ischemia. In addition, there is evidence that adenosine modulates high-energy phosphate utilization in either preconditioned or control, nonpreconditioned ischemic myocardium. The evidence regarding a signaling role of adenosine in preconditioning will be reviewed later in this chapter, whereas the immediate effect of adenosine on ischemic metabolism will be reviewed here.

In a recent study, we have assessed the effect of intracoronary adenosine on ischemic myocardial metabolism [55]. After perfusing one region of myocardium with adenosine and a separate region with adenosine-free buffer, blocks of adenosine treated and untreated myocardium from the same heart were subjected to total ischemia at 37°C in vitro. The rates of metabolism were compared based on metabolite content in samples from these myocardial blocks during 90 minutes of ischemia. Regional adenosine treatment slowed myocardial metabolism (Figure 7) to an extent comparable to that induced by ischemic preconditioning in the same test system [29]. In a subsequent study [56] we observed that when the selective A_1 adenosine antagonist BW-1433 was infused with the same concentration of adenosine, the energy-sparing effects of adenosine were abolished, supporting the hypothesis that adenosine mediates its protective effects through the A_1 re-

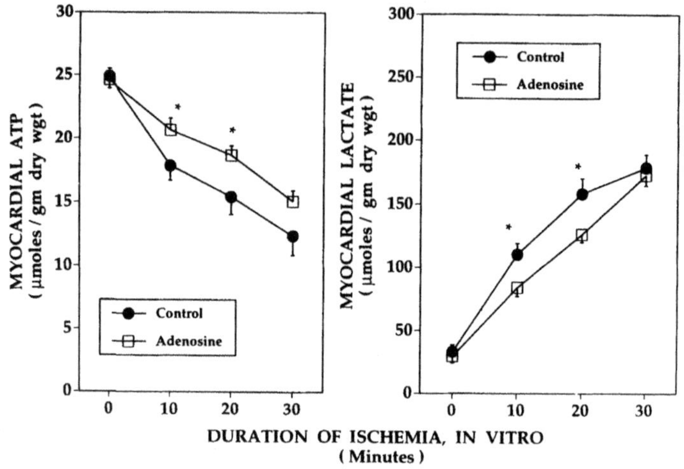

Figure 7. Effect of intracoronary adenosine infusion on myocardial content of adenosine triphosphate (ATP; **left**) and lactate (**right**) during in vitro total myocardial ischemia. Adenosine significantly slowed the rate of ATP depletion and of lactate accumulation during the first 20 minutes of myocardial ischemia. $P \leq 0.05$. Reprinted with permission from Vander Heide [55].

ceptor. In addition, pretreatment with the A_1 antagonist alone accelerated ATP depletion and lactate accumulation, suggesting that endogenous adenosine, acting through A_1 receptors, may be important in modulating ischemic energy demand. These results are consistent with the hypothesis that the known energy-slowing effects of ischemic preconditioning are mediated by adenosine produced during ischemia.

If adenosine produced during ischemia mediates the preconditioning effect, either more adenosine must be produced during ischemia in preconditioned myocardium, or preconditioned myocardium must be more sensitive to the available adenosine. In this regard, it recently has been reported that more adenosine is released following ischemia of preconditioned vs. virgin canine myocardium [57], and it has been proposed, based on results from isolated hypoxic cardiac myocytes, that this is related to a protein kinase C-mediated activation of 5′-nucleotidase [58]. On the contrary, other studies have shown that the amount of adenosine present during the test episode of ischemia is most likely *decreased* rather than increased in preconditioned vs. control myocardium [59,60]. For example, direct measurement of interstitial adenosine concentration during ischemia, using microdialysis probes, has shown less rather than more adenosine in ischemic myocardium after preconditioning [59].

Adenosine produced during the preconditioning episodes of ischemia either is washed out to the systemic circulation or utilized by the salvage pathway of adenine nucleotide synthesis for repletion of the adenine nucle-

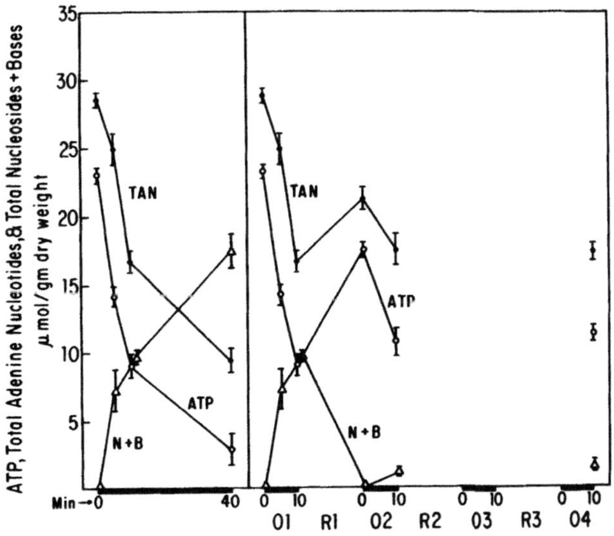

Figure 8. Myocardial adenosine triphosphate (ATP), total adenine nucleotide pool (TAN), and total pool of nucleosides and bases (N + B) during 40 minutes of continuous ischemia (**left**) and during 40 minutes of cumulative ischemia with intermittent reperfusion (**right**). Ten minutes of ischemia resulted in loss of 60% of the ATP and 40% of the adenine nucleotide pool. Reperfusion for 20 minutes then resulted in only partial repletion of ATP. Nevertheless, no cumulative loss of ATP occurred during three additional 10-minute episodes of ischemia. This is explained by a slower rate of ATP depletion in the later episodes. Note also that production of nucleosides and bases, the catabolites of adenine nucleotides, was substantial in the first ischemic episode but was markedly inhibited in later episodes. Reprinted with permission from Reimer et al. [60].

otide pool during reperfusion. During the subsequent episode of ischemia, the adenosine concentration is small because ATP breakdown to ADP is slowed, thereby also slowing catabolism of ADP to AMP and thence to adenosine. This, in turn, markedly reduces the accumulation of the nucleosides and bases, which result from the degradation of adenosine (Figure 8) [60]. Thus, if adenosine produced during the sustained test episode of ischemia causes greater metabolic slowing in preconditioned myocardium than in control myocardium, the effect must be mediated by much lower concentrations of adenosine. It follows that either more adenosine receptors must have become available or those available have become more sensitive to the smaller quantities of adenosine produced during the sustained ischemic episode. The hypothesis that adenosine produced during an initial episode of ischemia serves as a signal leading to reduced ischemic energy metabolism is discussed later in this chapter.

To better understand how adenosine might mediate the energy-sparing effects of ischemic preconditioning, it is necessary to review briefly what has been learned in recent years about adenosine receptors and the metabolic effects of adenosine receptor activation [61–64]. Adenosine receptors have been divided into at least two separate subgroups, A_1 and A_2, which have unique biologic and pharmacological profiles [65].

Adenosine A_1 receptors and pertussis toxin-sensitive G proteins

Activation of adenosine A_1 receptors has many effects, which differ among different regions of the heart and among different cell types. In ventricular myocardium, the actions are mediated primarily through coupling to guanine nucleotide regulatory proteins, specifically the inhibitory subtype (G_i proteins). Through this pathway, adenosine A_1 receptors couple to a variety of effector systems, including adenylate cyclase, phospholipase A_2 and C, potassium channels, calcium channels, guanylate cyclase, and the sodium–calcium exchange system [66–68]. Of the many effector systems to which adenosine A_1 receptor stimulation is coupled, the most clearly documented effects are inhibition of adenylate cyclase and activation of ATP-sensitive potassium channels [68]. In both isolated ventricular myocytes and intact ventricular myocardium, adenosine has been shown to inhibit adenylate cyclase (as measured by decreased levels of cAMP) [69,70]. Since cAMP activates a large number of effector proteins, inhibition of adenylate cyclase by adenosine could secondarily have profound metabolic (including energy-sparing) effects. Moreover, since adrenergic stimulation results in activation of adenylate cyclase, the inhibition of adenylate cyclase by adenosine can be considered to be an antiadrenergic effect [71–73]. For example, adenosine reduces calcium channel current in myocardium previously stimulated by beta-adrenergic agents [74,75]. Activation of the ATP-sensitive potassium channel [76] also could result in an energy-sparing effect. Among other actions, activation of this channel hyperpolarizes aerobic myocardium, thereby shortening the plateau phase of the action potential. Shortening of the action potential may, in turn, reduce inward calcium current through voltage-dependent calcium channels and thereby reduce energy demands for attempted contraction and maintenance of overall cellular calcium homeostasis.

In addition to direct actions on myocytes, adenosine has been shown to modulate noradrenaline release from nerve endings through a presynaptic mechanism [77–79]. Activation of A_1 receptors present on sympathetic nerve terminals results in an inhibition of exocytotic norepinephrine release that occurs during the early phase of myocardial ischemia [79,80]. Inhibition of norepinephrine release would lower interstitial catecholamine levels, which in turn would decrease adrenergic stimulation of the myocyte.

Blockade of G_i protein activity by pertussis toxin has been shown to inhibit the protective effect of adenosine in ischemic rat hearts [81] and to prevent ischemic preconditioning in rabbit hearts [82], providing support for the hypothesis that ischemic preconditioning is mediated through activation of the adenosine A_1 receptor coupled to a G_i protein. Involvement of a G_i protein also is supported by the observation in rabbits that preconditioning can be mimicked by the M_2 muscarinic agonist, carbachol, which also is coupled to the G_i protein, although not via the adenosine A_1 receptor [82].

Adenosine A_2 receptors

In myocardium, adenosine A_2 receptors are located primarily in the endothelium and vascular smooth muscle of the coronary vasculature [61]. Thus, adenosine A_2 receptors in the heart are thought to be important primarily in mediating the vasodilatory actions of adenosine [61,64]. However, recent data have suggested that A_2 receptors may be present on ventricular myocytes in some species [83]. In contrast to A_1 receptors, A_2 receptors stimulate adenylate cyclase through a stimulatory G protein, G_s. Thus, activation of A_2 receptors on ischemic myocytes would likely increase, rather than decrease, energy demand.

ATP sensitive K^+ channels

Another hyothesis to explain the cardioprotective effects of ischemic preconditioning involves ATP-dependent K^+ (K^+_{ATP}) channels. It has been proposed that preconditioning may cause increased activity of these channels by increasing the number that remain open after preconditioning, or by more rapidly opening more channels during a subsequent episode of ischemia [84]. One way in which greater K^+_{ATP} channel activity might be protective is through a shortening of the plateau phase of the action potential and consequent shortening of the duration of inward flux of Ca^{++}. This would reduce the ATP required to support Ca^{++} cycling.

Evidence supporting this K^+_{ATP} channel hypothesis of preconditioning comes from studies in dogs. Glibenclamide (an inhibitor of the K^+_{ATP} channel), when administered either before or after brief ischemia, abolished the protective effect of ischemic preconditioning [84]. Moreover, the K^+_{ATP} channel openers nicorandil and pinacidil have been reported to have antiischemic properties in virgin myocardium [85,86]. However, the aforementioned positive results from dogs regarding the role of K^+_{ATP} channels in preconditioning are contradicted by results from rabbits and rats [87,88]. In the latter studies, glibenclamide did not abolish the protective effect of preconditioning. It should be noted that the K^+ channel hypothesis and the adenosine hypothesis are not mutually exclusive, since activation of A_1 adenosine receptors is one of the means available to open the potassium channel [76].

Antiadrenergic effects

Norepinephrine is released from sympathetic nerve endings during the first few minutes of ischemia [79,80]. The resulting stimulation of beta-adrenergic receptors on ventricular myocytes activates adenylate cyclase and thereby accelerates a variety of energy utilizing reactions [89]. Thus, either a reduction in norepinephrine release from sympathetic nerve endings to the my-

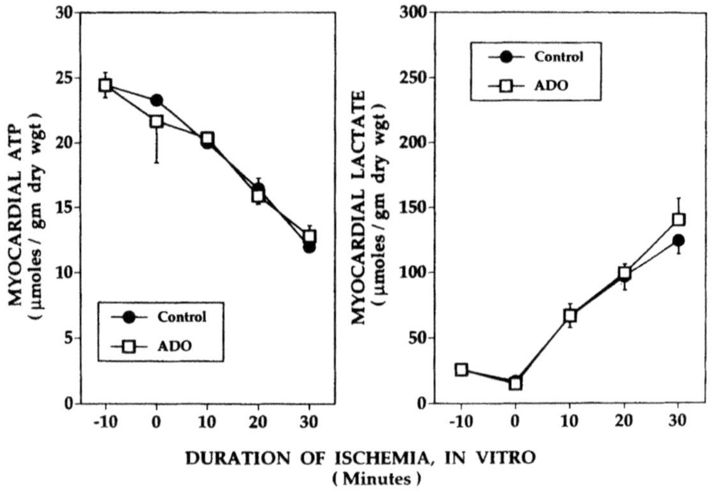

Figure 9. Effect of adenosine infusion on myocardial content of adenosine triphosphate (ATP); (**left**) and lactate (**right**) during in vitro total ischemia in hearts from dogs depleted of endogenous catecholamines by pretreatment 24 hours earlier with reserpine. Adenosine did not further slow the rate of ATP depletion or lactate accumulation compared to control tissue from the same hearts. Reprinted with permission from Vander Heide et al. [56].

ocardial interstitium, or a reduced myocyte responsiveness to norepinephrine could having an energy-sparing effect.

Since adenosine A_1 receptor stimulation is capable of inhibiting both norepinephrine release from nerve endings [77–79] and cAMP-dependent energy-utilizing reactions, adenosine may retard catecholamine-mediated energy utilization during the early phase of myocardial ischemia.

If the energy-sparing effect of adenosine is mediated through an antiadrenergic mechanism, elimination of myocardial catecholamines before ischemia should have the same energy-sparing effect as adenosine, and adenosine should have no additional effect in catecholamine-depleted hearts. To test this hypothesis, we recently have studied the effect of adenosine on energy metabolism in dogs pretreated with reserpine, which depletes nerve terminals of their norepinephrine stores. Indeed, ATP depletion and lactate accumulation in control myocardium from reserpine-treated dogs occurred at a rate similar to that in adenosine-treated myocardium from untreated dogs [55], and adenosine had no additional effect in reserpine-treated hearts (Figure 9) [56]. These results are consistent with the hypothesis that adenosine slows ischemic metabolism through an antiadrenergic effect.

The principal evidence against an antiadrenergic mechanism of ischemic preconditioning is the lack of efficacy of beta-blocking agents in limiting myocardial infarct size in several experimental models [90,91]. However, beta-blocking drugs are competitive inhibitors of the beta-adrenergic receptor, and it is not known whether nontoxic doses of beta blockers yield sufficient myocardial concentrations to block the effect of the locally large concentration of norepinephrine that can be released in ischemic myocardium. In addition, selective blockade of beta receptors does not inhibit alpha$_1$-adrenergic receptors, which are known to be present in mammalian myocardium. Activation of alpha$_1$ receptors may have positive inotropic effects when beta-adrenergic receptors are blocked [89]. Alpha$_1$-receptor stimulation activates phospholipase C (PLC) through a G-protein-mediated mechanism. Enhanced function of PLC increases production of the second messengers inositol triphosphate (IP_3) and diacylglycerol (DAG), which, in turn, increase the release of Ca^{++} from intracellular stores and activate protein kinase C. The net effect of PLC activation is increased contractility and increased intracellular calcium cycling [89].

Unifying hypotheses regarding pathways through which energy metabolism may be slowed in preconditioned myocardium

The several hypotheses currently under consideration are summarized diagrammatically in Figure 10. One or more proximal mechanisms may lead to

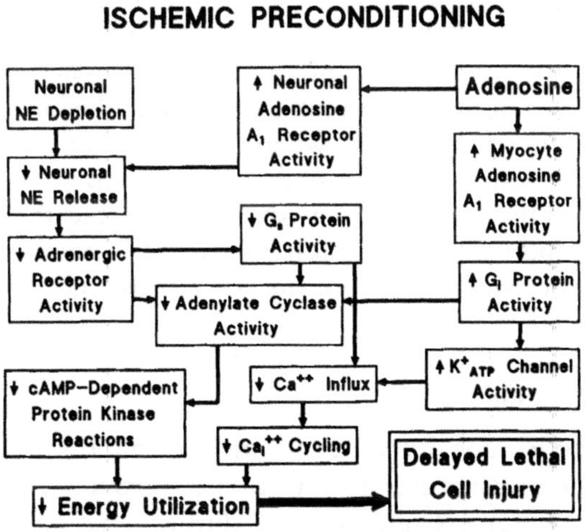

Figure 10. Summary of currently popular hypotheses that may explain both the energy-sparing and infarct-limiting effects of ischemic preconditioning. Energy-utilizing reactions include cellular calcium cycling and a variety of metabolic processes modulated by cAMP-dependent protein kinases. These processes are modulated by activation of a variety of sarcolemmal receptors, including alpha- and beta-adrenergic receptors, muscarinic receptors, and the A_1 and A_2 adenosine receptors, which in turn control the relative activities of inhibitory (G_i) and stimulatory (G_s) guanine nucleotide regulatory proteins (G proteins). Ischemic preconditioning hypothetically may reduce ischemic metabolism by acting at one or more of these interacting pathways and regulatory steps (see also Table 1). Hypothetical signals through which ischemic metabolism might be modulated include activation of adenosine A_1 receptors on either myocytes or cardiac nerve terminals, or modulation of K^+_{ATP} channel activity.

a final common pathway through which preconditioning mediates energy-sparing and cellular protective effects. As illustrated on this diagram, some of the proximal mechanisms discussed above are not mutually exclusive. Which of these or other pathways are most important in mediating preconditioning is uncertain. In addition, the mechanisms through which these pathways may be altered by a brief episode of ischemia remain unknown.

WHAT IS THE SIGNAL PRODUCED BY ISCHEMIA THROUGH WHICH THIS REDUCED ENERGY DEMAND IS ACHIEVED?

Adenosine

Recent evidence, primarily from rabbits, has shown that adenosine receptor activation, specifically adenosine A_1 receptor stimulation, is capable of producing profound cardioprotection, similar in degree to that induced by ischemic preconditioning [92,93]. For example, either a brief intracoronary infusion of adenosine or intravenous infusion of potent A_1 adenosine receptor agonists, such as N^6-phenyl-2R-isopropyl adenosine (PIA) or 2-chloro-N^6-cyclophenyladenosine (CPA), was shown to mimick the reduction in infarct size achieved by a short period of ischemia [92]. Moreover, it has been shown that infusion of a nonselective adenosine receptor antagonist (PD-115,119), either before or after a short preconditioning episode of ischemia, abolishes the protective effect of ischemic preconditioning [93].

As discussed earlier, adenosine might mediate the energy-sparing and cardioprotective effects of preconditioning. However, the likelihood that adenosine is washed out of the tissue before the onset of subsequent ischemic episodes, coupled with observations that less adenosine is produced during the test episode, is more consistent with the hypothesis that activation of the A_1 adenosine receptor prior to the test episode of ischemia serves as a switch to reduce ischemic energy metabolism. How this may be achieved is presently unknown.

Adrenergic modulation

As discussed above, one hypothetical mechanism through which preconditioning may cause myocardial protection is through a reduction either in the amount of norepinephrine released during a second (test) episode of ischemia or in myocyte responsiveness to beta-receptor stimulation. This might occur through several mechanisms. For example, as discussed earlier, activation of adenosine A_1 receptors on sympathetic nerve terminals during preconditioning might inhibit norepinephrine release during subsequent ischemia. Alternatively, partial depletion of norepinephrine might occur during preconditioning due to washout rather than reuptake of norepinephrine during reperfusion. If so, less norepinephrine would be available for release during the second episode of ischemia. In addition, ischemic preconditioning might result in a downregulation or inactivation of myocyte beta-receptors (i.e., by phosphorylation). To date, however, there is little direct evidence to support or refute these hypotheses.

A related but different proposal is that myocardial protection may result from a preceding alpha-adrenergic stimulation during a preconditioning protocol [94]. This hypothesis is supported by the observation that preconditioning against contractile dysfunction could be prevented in isolated rat hearts by administration of an alpha-receptor blocker [94]. Further support for a protective effect induced by preliminary alpha-adrenergic stimulation has been obtained in rabbits, in which pretreatment with tyramine, an agent which induces release of norepinephrine from sympathetic nerve terminals, mimicked the effect of preconditioning, i.e., resulted in smaller myocardial infarcts after a test episode of ischemia and reperfusion [95]. Moreover, this beneficial effect of tyramine was abolished by simultaneous administration of BE 2254, an antagonist of the alpha$_1$-adrenergic receptor. However, in the same study, BE 2254 pretreatment did not prevent the limitation of infarct size by ischemic preconditioning, casting doubt on the hypothesis that the mechanism of ischemic preconditioning is explained simply by the protection induced by preliminary alpha-adrenergic stimulation.

Changes in gene expression

It has been proposed that a brief episode of ischemia might induce the transcription of new mRNA and subsequent synthesis of one or more protective proteins, akin to the heat shock response, that might protect the myocardium from ischemic cell injury. Several observations support this possibility. First, heat shock in rats [3] and rabbits [4] was reported to have a cardioprotective effect against a myocardial ischemic insult 24 hours later. Secondly, a nonlethal episode (10 or 15 minutes) of ischemia in dogs was found to induce the synthesis of mRNA for stress proteins, detectable during reperfusion as early as 60 minutes after the ischemic insult [96].

However, it seems unlikely that the time course of such a mechanism could be consistent with the general biology of preconditioning: (1) The protein message presumably would have to be produced within a few minutes after reperfusion and (2) the message would have to be lost or countermanded after 90–120 minutes of reperfusion (even though the quantities of the known stress proteins have been observed to continue increasing much beyond these times [1,97,98]). Indeed, recent evidence has cast doubt on the hypothesis. For example, exposure of canine myocardium to regional hyperthermia 1 hour before a 60-minute coronary occlusion did not limit myocardial infarct size, even though synthesis of mRNA for stress proteins was detected before the onset of ischemia [99]. In other studies, neither inhibition of transcription of RNA from DNA using actinomycin D nor inhibition of protein translation from the RNA message with cycloheximide attenuated the protective effect of ischemic preconditioning in rabbits [10,100]. These studies suggest that preconditioning is not dependent on rapid synthesis of a new class of proteins. However, these studies do not rule out the possibility that translocation of preformed "shuttle proteins," including stress proteins, might play a role in the preconditioning response (see Chapter 6).

Free radical-mediated injury

The possibility that ischemic preconditioning might be a favorable consequence of oxygen-derived free radical mediated injury was suggested as a corollary of the "stunning mediates preconditioning" hypothesis [101]. Specifically, it was proposed that (1) because substantial evidence implicates oxygen-derived free radicals as contributory causes of stunning [47], and (2) if stunning mediates preconditioning, then free radical injury could paradoxically mediate the protective effect of preconditioning. Although superoxide dismutase (SOD) plus catalase substantially attenuates the severe stunning resulting from a 15-minute episode of ischemia, this anti-free-radical treatment did not further attenuate the mild degree of stunning observed following four 5-minute episodes of ischemia [102]. However, it did abolish the protective effect of preconditioning in 5 of the 11 dogs studied. The explanation for this non-uniform effect of treatment with SOD plus catalase remains unexplained. Moreover, this hypothesis could not be confirmed in a study in rabbits [11], in which anti-free-radical therapy had no detrimental effect on ischemic preconditioning.

Unifying hypotheses

At present, the signal(s) through which myocardial energy metabolism is reduced by ischemic preconditioning is unknown. From the preceding discussion, several signals are hypothetically possible and are included in Table 4. Establishing the signal and the altered metabolic pathways that affect the preconditioning response remains the major challenge to students of this endogenous cardioprotective phenomenon.

Table 4. Hypothetical signals and metabolic pathways through which myocardial energy metabolism may be reduced by ischemic preconditioning

1.	Decreased neuronal release of norepinephrine
2.	Decreased adrenergic (alpha or beta) receptor expression or sensitivity to norepinephrine stimulation
3.	Increased interstitial adenosine concentration during ischemia
4.	Increased A_1 and/or decreased A_2 receptor expression or sensitivity to a second exposure to adenosine
5.	Increased G_i or decreased G_s sensitivity to activation
6.	Increased K^+ channel flux and/or decreased Ca^{++} channel flux
7.	Reduced activity of one or more myocyte ATPases

REFERENCES

1. Currie RW. 1987. Effects of ischemia and perfusion temperature on the synthesis of stress-induced (heat shock) proteins in isolated and perfused rat hearts. J Mol Cell Cardiol 19:795–808.
2. Yellon DM, Latchman DS. 1992. Stress proteins and myocardial protection. J Mol Cell Cardiol 24:113–124.
3. Currie RW, Karmazyn M, Kloc M, Mailer K. 1988. Heat-shock response is associated with enhanced postischemic ventricular recovery. Circ Res 63:543–549.
4. Yellon DM, Pasini E, Cargnoni A, Marber MS, Latchman DS, Ferrari R. 1992. The protective role of heat stress in the ischaemic and reperfused rabbit myocardium. J Mol Cell Cardiol 24:895–907.
5. Walker DM, Pasini E, Kucukoglu S, Marber MS, Iliodromitis E, Ferrari R, Yellon DM. 1993. Heat stress limits infarct size in the isolated blood and buffer perfused rabbit heart. Cardiovasc Res, in press.
6. Donnelly TJ, Sievers RE, Vissern FLJ, Welch WJ, Wolfe CL. 1992. Heat shock protein induction in rat hearts. A role for improved myocardial salvage after ischemia and reperfusion? Circulation 85:769–778.
7. Murry CE, Jennings RB, Reimer KA. 1986. Preconditioning with ischemia: A delay of lethal cell injury in ischemic myocardium. Circulation 74:1124–1136.
8. Li GC, Vasquez JA, Gallagher KP, Lucchesi BR. 1990. Myocardial protection with preconditioning. Circulation 82:609–619.
9. Schott RJ, Rohmann S, Braun ER, Schaper W. 1990. Ischemic preconditioning reduces infarct size in swine myocardium. Circ Res 66:1133–1142.
10. Thornton JD, Striplin S, Liu GS, Swafford A, Stanley AH, Van Winkle DM, Downey JM. 1990. Inhibition of protein synthesis does not block myocardial protection afforded by preconditioning. Am J Physiol (Heart Circ Physiol) 259:H1822–H1825.
11. Iwamoto T, Miura T, Adachi T, Noto T, Ogowa T, Tsuchida A, Iimura O. 1991. Myocardial infarct size-limiting effect of ischemic preconditioning was not attenuated by oxygen free-radical scavengers in the rabbit. Circulation 83:1015–1022.
12. Cohen MV, Liu GS, Downey JM. 1991. Preconditioning causes improved wall motion as well as smaller infarcts after transient coronary occlusion in rabbits. Circulation 84:341–349.
13. Li Y, Whittaker P, Kloner RA. 1992. The transient nature of the effect of ischemic preconditioning on myocardial infarct size and ventricular arrhythmia. Am Heart J 123: 346–353.
14. Li Y, Kloner RA. 1992. Cardioprotective effects of ischaemic "preconditioning" are not mediated by prostanoids. Cardiovasc Res 26:226–231.
15. Yellon DM, Alkhulaifi AM, Browne EE, Pugsley WB. 1992. Ischemic preconditioning limits infarct size in the rat heart. Cardiovasc Res 26:983–987.
16. Murry CE, Richard VJ, Reimer KA, Jennings RB. 1990. Ischemic preconditioning slows energy metabolism and delays ultrastructural damage during a sustained ischemic episode. Circ Res 66:913–931.
17. Lowe JE, Jennings RB, Reimer KA. 1979. Cardiac rigor mortis in dogs. J Mol Cell Cardiol 11:1017–1031.
18. Kagawa Y. 1984. Proton motive ATP synthesis. In Energetics, L Ernster, ed. Elsevier, Amsterdam, pp. 149–186.
19. Rouslin W, Erickson JL, Solaro RJ. 1986. Effects of oligomycin and acidosis on rates of ATP depletion in ischemic heart muscle. Am J Physiol 250:H503–H508.
20. Jennings RB, Reimer KA, Steenbergen C, Jr. 1991.. Effect of inhibition of the mitochondrial ATPase on net myocardial ATP in total ischemia. J Mol Cell Cardiol 230:1383–1395.
21. Pullman ME, Monroy GC. 1963. A naturally occuring inhibitor of mitochondrial adenosine triphosphatase. J Biol Chem 238:3762–3769.
22. Neely JR, Morgan HE. 1974. Relationship between carbohydrate and lipid metabolism and the energy balance of heart muscle. Ann Rev Physiol 36:413–459.
23. Mochizuki S, Neely JR. 1979. Control of glyceraldehyde-3-phosphate dehydrogenase in cardiac muscle. J Mol Cell Cardiol 11:221–236.

24. Jones RN, Reimer KA, Hill ML, Jennings RB. 1982. Effect of hypothermia on changes in high-energy phosphate production and utilization in total ischemia. J Mol Cell Cardiol 14(Suppl 3):123–130.
25. Reimer KA, Hill ML, Jennings RB. 1981. Prolonged depletion of ATP and of the adenine nucleotide pool due to delayed resynthesis of adenine nucleotides following reversible myocardial ischemic injury in dogs. J Mol Cell Cardiol 13:229–239.
26. Swain JL, Sabina RL, Hines JJ, Greenfield JC, Jr, Holmes EW. 1984. Repetitive episodes of brief ischaemia (12 min) do not produce a cumulative depletion of high energy phosphate compounds. Cardiovasc Res 18:264–269.
27. Basuk WL, Reimer KA, Jennings RB. 1986. Effect of repetitive brief episodes of ischemia on cell volume, electrolytes and ultrastructure. J Am Coll Cardiol 8(Suppl A):A33–A41.
28. Swain JL, Sabina RL, McHale PA, Greenfield JC, Jr, Holmes EW. 1982. Prolonged myocardial adenine nucleotide depletion after brief ischemia in the open-chest dog. Am J Physiol 242:H818–826.
29. Jennings RB, Murry CE, Reimer KA. 1991. Energy metabolism in preconditioned and control myocardium: Effect of total ischemia. J Mol Cell Cardiol 23:1449–1458.
30. Reimer KA, Jennings RB. 1991. Cardiac metabolic responses to ischemia. In Textbook of Internal Medicine, 2nd ed. W Kelley, ed. J.B. Lippincott, Philadelphia, pp. 1089–1094.
31. Yamamoto H, Tomoike H, Shimokawa H, Nabeyama S, Nakamura M. 1984. Development of collateral function with repetitive coronary occlusion in a canine model reduces myocardial reactive hyperemia in the absence of significant coronary stenosis. Circ Res 55:623–632.
32. Murry CE, Richard VJ, Jennings RB, Reimer KA. 1991. Myocardial protection is lost before contractile function recovers from ischemic preconditioning. Am J Physiol (Heart Circ Physiol) 260:H796–H804.
33. Ichihara K, Abiko Y. 1984. Rebound recovery of myocardial creatine phosphate with reperfusion after ischemia. Am Heart J 108:1594–1597.
34. Wyatt DA, Edmunds MC, Rubio R, Berne RM, Lasley RD, Mentzer RM, Jr. 1989. Adenosine stimulates glycolytic flux in isolated perfused rat hearts by A_1-adenosine receptors. Am J Physiol 257(6):H1952–H1957.
35. Neely JR, Whitmer JT, Rovetto MJ. 1975. Effect of coronary blood flow on glycolytic flux and intracellular pH in isolated rat hearts. Circ Res 37:733–741.
36. Wolfe CL, Sievers RE, Vissern FLJ, Donnelly, TJ. 1993. Loss of myocardial protection after preconditioning correlates with the time course of glycogen recovery within the preconditioned segment. Circulation 87:881–892.
37. Omar BA, Hanson AK, Bose SK, McCord JM. 1991. Reperfusion with pyruvate eliminates ischemic preconditioning in isolated rabbit heart: An apparent role for enhanced glycolysis. Coron Artery Dis 2:799–804.
38. Fralix TA, Steenbergen C, Jr, London RE, Murphy E. 1992. Metabolic substrates can alter postischemic recovery in preconditioned ischemic heart. Am J Physiol 263:C17–C23.
39. Liu GS, Downey JM. 1992. Preconditioning protects against myocardial infarction equally well with pyruvate or glucose containing reperfusate. J Mol Cell Cardiol 24(Suppl I):S93 (abstr).
40. Alkhulaifi AM, Pugsley WB, Yellon DM. 1993. The influence of the time period between ischemic preconditioning and prolonged ischemia on myocardial protection. Cardioscience, in press.
41. Nao BS, McClanahan TB, Groh MA, Schott RJ, Gallagher KP. 1990. The time limit of effective ischemic preconditioning in dogs. Circulation 88(Suppl III):III271 (abstr).
42. Vander Heide RS, Hill ML, Steenbergen C, Jr, Reimer KA, Jennings RB. 1991. Effect of reversible ischemia on mitochondrial ATPase activity in canine myocardium. Circulation 84(Suppl 4):II192 (abstr).
43. Schwertzmann K, Pedersen PL. 1981. Proton-adenosinetriphosphatase complex of rat liver mitochondria: Effect of energy state on its interaction with the adenosinetriphosphate inhibitory peptide. Biochemistry 20:6305–6311.
44. Rouslin W, Pullman ME. 1987. Protonic inhibition of the mitochondrial adenosine 5′-triphosphatase in ischemic cardiac muscle. Reversible binding of the ATPase inhibitor protein to the mitochondrial ATPase during ischemia. J Mol Cell Cardiol 19:661–668.
45. Rouslin W, Broge CW, Grupp IL. 1990. ATP depletion and mitochondrial functional loss

during ischemia in slow and fast heart-rate hearts. Am J Physiol 259:H1759–H1766.
46. Braunwald E, Kloner RA. 1982. The stunned myocardium: Prolonged, postischemic ventricular dysfunction. Circulation 66:1146–1149.
47. Bolli R. 1990. Mechanism of myocardial stunning. Circulation 82:723–738.
48. Schroder E, Kieso RA, Laughlin D, Schroder M, Meng R, Kerber RE. 1987. Altered response of reperfused myocardium to repeated coronary occlusion in dogs. J Am Coll Cardiol 10:898–905.
49. Schwarz ER, Mohri M, Sack S, Arras M, Schaper W. 1992. Preconditioning by ischemia lasts only for 30 minutes and is inhibited by adenosine antagonists. J Mol Cell Cardiol 24(Suppl I):S93 (abstr).
50. Miura T, Goto M, Urabe K, Enoh A, Shimamoto K, Iimura O. 1991. Does myocardial stunning contribute to infarct size limitation by ischemic preconditioning? Circulation 84:2504–2512.
51. Matsuda M, Catena TG, Vander Heide RS, Jennings RB, Reimer KA. 1993. Cardiac protection by ischemic preconditioning is not mediated by myocardial stunning. Cardiovasc Res 27:585–592.
52. Jennings RB, Murry CE, Reimer KA. 1991. Preconditioning myocardium with ischemia. Cardiovasc Drugs Ther 5:933–938.
53. Rohmann S, Scott RJ, Harting J, Schaper W. 1991. Ischemic preconditioning is not a function of stunned myocardium. J Mol Cell Cardiol 23(Suppl V):S71 (abstr).
54. Ovize M, Przyklenk K, Hale SL, Kloner RA. 1992. Preconditioning does not attenuate myocardial stunning. Circulation 85:2247–2254.
55. Vander Heide RS, Reimer KA, Jennings RB. 1993. Adenosine slows ischemic metabolism in canine myocardium in vitro: Relationship to ischemic preconditioning. Cardiovasc. Res, in press.
56. Vander Heide RS, Reimer KA, Jennings RB. 1992. Adenosine mimicks ischemic preconditioning in its effects on ischemic myocardial metabolism—possible role of catecholamines. J Mol Cell Cardiol 24(Suppl I):S64 (abstr).
57. Kitakaze M, Hori M, Takashima S, Sato H, Inoue M, Kamada T. 1993. Ischemic preconditioning increases adenosine release and 5′ nucleotidase activity during myocardial ischemia and reperfusion: Implications for myocardial salvage. Circulation 87:208–215.
58. Kitakaze M, Kitabatake A. 1991. Increased 5′ nucleotidase activity caused by protein kinase C enhances adenosine production in hypoxic cardiomyocytres. Circulation 84(Suppl 2): II620 (abstr).
59. Dorheim T, Mentzer RD, Van Wylen D. 1991. Preconditioning reduces interstitial fluid purine metabolites during prolonged myocardial ischemia. Circulation 84(Suppl 2):II191 (abstr).
60. Reimer KA, Murry CE, Yamasawa I, Hill ML, Jennings RB. 1986. Four brief periods of myocardial ischemia cause no cumulative ATP loss or necrosis. Am J Physiol 251:H1306–H1315.
61. Belardinelli L, Linden J, Berne RM. 1989. The cardiac effects of adenosine. Prog Cardiovasc Dis 32:73–97.
62. Pantely GA, Bristow JD. 1990. Adenosine. Renewed interest in an old drug. Circulation 82:1854–1856.
63. Mullane KM. 1992. Myocardial preconditioning. Part of the adenosine revival. Circulation 85:845–847.
64. Ely SW, Berne RM. 1992. Protective effects of adenosine in myocardial ischemia. Circulation 85:893–904.
65. Burnstock G. 1978. A basis for distinguishing two types of purinergic receptors. In Cell Membrane Receptors for Drugs and Hormones: A Multidiscipilinary Approach, L Bolis, RW Straub, eds. Raven Press, New York, pp. 107–118.
66. Olsson RA, Pearson JD. 1990. Cardiovascular purinoceptors. Physiol Rev 70:761–845.
67. Neer EJ, Clapham DE. 1992. Signal transduction through G proteins in the cardiac myocyte. Trends Cardiovasc Med 2:6–11.
68. Stiles GL. 1991. Adenosine receptors: Physiological regulation and biochemical mechanisms. News Physiol Sci 6:161–165.
69. Belardinelli L, Isenberg G. 1983. Actions of adenosine and isoproterenol on isolated mammalian ventricular myocytes. Circ Res 53:287–297.

70. Isenberg G, Belardinelli L. 1984. Ionic basis for the antagonism between adenosine and isoproterenol on isolated mammalian ventricular myocytes. Circ Res 55:309–325.
71. Romano FD, Naimi TS, Dobson JG, Jr. 1991. Adenosine attenuation of catecholamine-enhanced contractility of rat heart in vivo. Am J Physiol (Heart Circ Physiol) 260:H1635–H1639.
72. Romano FD, Dobson JG, Jr. 1990. Adenosine modulates β-adrenergic signal transduction in guinea pig heart ventricular membranes. J Mol Cell Cardiol 22:1359–1370.
73. Schrader J, Gerlach E, Baumann G. 1979. Sites and mode of action of adenosine in the heart. II. Ventricular myocardium. In Physiological and Regulatory Functions of Adenosine and Adenine Nucletides, HP Baer, GI Drummond, eds. Raven Press, New York, pp. 137–144.
74. Kato M, Yamaguchi H, Ochi R. 1990. Mechanism of adenosine-induced inhibition of calcium current in guinea pig ventricular cells. Circ Res 67:1134–1141.
75. Isenberg G, Cerbai E, Klockner U. 1987. Ionic channels and adenosine in isolated heart cells. In Topics and Perspectives in Adenosine Research, E Gerlach, BF Becker, eds. Springer-Verlag, Berlin, pp. 324–335.
76. Kirsch GE, Codina J, Birnbaumer L, Brown AM. 1990. Coupling of ATP-sensitive K^+ channels to A_1 receptors by G proteins in rat ventricular myocytes. Am J Physiol 259: H820–H826.
77. Fredholm BB, Hedquist P. 1980. Modulation of neuro-transmission by purine nucleotides and nucleosides. Biochem Pharmacol 29:1635–1643.
78. Wakade AR, Wakade TD. 1978. Inhibition of noradrenaline release by adenosine. J Physiol 282:35–49.
79. Schöming A. 1990. Catecholamines in myocardial ischemia. Systemic and cardiac release. Circulation 82(Suppl II):13–22.
80. Richardt G, Wass W, Kranzhofer R, Mayer E, Schöming A. 1987. Adenosine inhibits exocytotic release of endogenous noradrenaline in rat heart: A protective mechanism in early myocardial ischemia. Circ Res 61:117–123.
81. Lasley RD, Barakat O, Van Wylen GL, Mentzer RD. 1991. Pertussis toxin inhibits adenosine-mediated preservation of post-ischemic myocardial function. Circulation 84 (Suppl 2):II307 (abstr).
82. Thornton JD, Downey JM. 1991. G_i proteins are involved in preconditioning's protective effect. Circulation 84(Suppl II):II192 (abstr).
83. Liang BT. 1992. Atrium- and ventricle-specific expression of adenosine receptor subtypes: Functional and molecular evidence for a stimulatory adenosine receptor subtype on ventricular myocytes. J Mol Cell Cardiol 24(Suppl I):S63 (abstr).
84. Gross GJ, Auchampach JA. 1992. Blockade of ATP-sensitive potassium channels prevents myocardial preconditioning in dogs. Circulation 70:223–233.
85. Gross GJ, Pieper GM, Faber NE, Warltier DC, Hardman HF. 1989. Effects of nicorandil on coronary circulation and myocardial ischemia. Am J Cardiol 63:11J–17J.
86. Grover GJ, McCullough JR, Henry DE, Conder ML, Sleph PG. 1990. Anti-ischemic effects of the potassium channel activators pinacidil and cromakalim and the reversal of these effects with the potassium channel blocker glyburide. J Pharm Exp Ther 251:98–104.
87. Thornton JD, Downey JM. 1991. Blockade of ATP-sensitive potassium channels does not prevent preconditioning in the rabbit heart. Circulation 84(Suppl II):II432 (abstr).
88. Liu Y, Downey JM. 1992. Preconditioning protects against infarction in the rat heart. J Mol Cell Cardiol 24(Suppl 3):S5 (abstr).
89. Fleming JW, Wisler PL, Watanabe AM. 1992. Signal transduction by G proteins in cardiac tissues. Circulation 85:420–423.
90. Jennings RB, Reimer KA. 1979. Effect of beta adrenergic blockade on acute myocardial ischemic injury. In Modulation of Sympathetic Tone in the Treatment of Cardiovascular Diseases, F. Gross, ed. Hans Huber Publishers, Bern, Switzerland, pp. 103–116.
91. Hearse DJ, Yellon DM, Downey JM. 1986. Can beta blockers limit infarct size? Eur Heart J 7:925–930.
92. Thornton JD, Liu GS, Olsson RA, Downey JM. 1992. Intravenous pretreatment with A_1 selective adenosine analogs protects the heart against infarction. Circulation 85:659–665.
93. Liu GS, Thornton JD, Van Winkle DM, Stanley AWH, Olsson RA, Downey JM. 1991. Protection against infarction afforded by preconditioning is mediated by A_1 adenosine receptors in rabbit heart. Circulation 84:350–356.

94. Locke-Winter CR, Winter CB, Nelson DW, Bannerjee A. 1991. cAMP stimulation facilitates preconditioning against ischemia-reperfusion through norepinephrine and $alpha_1$ mechanisms. Circulation 84(Suppl II):II433 (abstr).
95. Thornton JD, Daly JF, Cohen MV, Downey JM. 1993. Catecholamines can induce adenosine receptor-mediated protection of the myocardium but do not participate in ischemic preconditioning in the rabbit. Circ Res, in press.
96. Fleischman KE, Brand T, Sharma HS, Duncker DJ, Sassen LMA, McFalls EO, Verdouw PD, Schaper W. 1990. Gene expression in a preconditioning model. Circulation 82(Suppl III):III464 (abstr).
97. Dillmann WH, Mehta HB, Barrieux A, Guth BD, Neeley WE, Ross J Jr. 1986. Ischemia of the dog heart induces the appearance of a cardiac mRNA coding for a protein with migration characteristics similar to heat-shock/stress protein 71. Circ Res 59:110–114.
98. Kucukoglu S, Iliodromites E, Van Winkle DM, Downery JM, Marber M, Heads R, Yellon DM. 1991. Protection by ischemic preconditioning appears independent of stress protein synthesis. J Mol Cell Cardiol 23(Suppl V):S71 (abstr).
99. Schott RJ, Nao BS, Strieter R, Groh M, Kunkee S, McClanahan T, Schaper W. 1990. Heat shock does not "precondition" canine myocardium. Circulation 82(Suppl III):III464 (abstr).
100. Kuckogku S, Ilidromitis E, Van Winkle D, Downey J, Marber M, Heads R, Yellon DM. 1991. Protection by ischaemic preconditioning appears independent of stress protein synthesis. J Mol Cell Cardiol 23(Suppl V):S73 (abstr).
101. Murry CE, Richard VJ, Jennings RB, Reimer KA. 1988. Preconditioning with ischemia: Is the protective effect mediated by free radical-induced myocardial stunning? Circulation 78(Suppl II):77 (abstr).
102. Murry CE, Richard VJ, Jennings RB, Reimer KA. 1989. Free radicals do not cause myocardial stunning after four 5 minute coronary occlusions. Circulation 80(Suppl II):296 (abstr).
103. Jennings RB, Reimer KA, Steenbergen C, Jr, Murry CE. 1987. Energy metabolism in myocardial ischemia and reperfusion. In Myocardial Ischemia, NS Dhalla, IR Innes, RE Beamish, eds. Boston A: Martinus Njhoff, pp. 185–189.
104. Jennings RB, Reimer KA. 1981. Lethal myocardial ischemic injury. Am J Pathol 102:241–255.

6. STRESS PROTEINS, HEAT STRESS, AND MYOCARDIAL PROTECTION

MICHAEL S. MARBER, RICHARD J. HEADS, and DEREK M. YELLON

INTRODUCTION

For the last two decades there has been an enormous effort to find therapeutic means of protecting the ischemic and reperfused myocardium. Numerous studies concentrated on finding and targeting specific pharmacological agents in an attempt to reduce experimental infarct size, with the ultimate clinical aim of limiting postinfarct morbidity and mortality [1,2]. Unfortunately such agents never came to the fore, and it was accepted that drugs may at best have the ability to delay ischemia/reperfusion injury without an appreciable effect on ultimate myocardial infarct size [3,4].

The failure to find specific "antiischemic" pharmacological agents has stimulated interest in the heart's adaptive responses and an investigation into the endogenous abilities of the heart to limit infarction. It is hoped that by understanding such cellular and molecular adaptation, *endogenous routes to myocardial protection* will be found, allowing future rational design and testing of specific agents that mimic these effects.

In this context both the phenomena of ischemic preconditioning [5] and heat stress [6] appear to increase cardiac defenses against ischemia and reperfusion. Ischemic preconditioning has been an area of intensive research, the results of which are presented in other chapters of this book. Although the protective benefits of whole-body heat stress have been well documented [6], the investigation of the role of stress proteins in this protection remains at an early stage, with a large number of experimental findings available only in a preliminary abstract form. The aim of this chapter is to review the evidence for stress protein involvement in ischemic preconditioning and to discuss the relationship between stress proteins, heat stress, and myocardial protection.

DEFINING THE TERMINOLOGY

Thermotolerance and crosstolerance

Hyperthermia induces the synthesis, in the heart and other tissue, of a small group of proteins known as the heat shock or stress proteins (hsp's). The cells that are subjected to such a stress and that accumulate stress proteins acquire a transient resistance to further episodes of thermal stress [7–9]. The dependence of this phenomenon of *acquired thermotolerance* on individual stress proteins has been demonstrated (i) using anti-sense RNA [10] to specifically hybridize with, and prevent the translation of, heat stress protein mRNA and (ii) by producing cell lines with heat stress protein gene deletions [11]. Conversely, a "genetically engineered" increase in the basal expression of a particular stress protein can confer themotolerance [12]. Similarly, and perhaps of greater interest, is the observation that stress protein induced by one stress can protect against a differing subsequent stress. Hence, stress proteins synthesised as result of exposure to ethanol and sodium arsenite are able to confer themotolerance [13]. This phenomenon, which is related to *acquired thermotolerance*, is known as *crosstolerance*. Thus, logic would dictate that if a particular nonthermal stress is associated with stress protein production, then tissue with thermally preelevated stress protein should have an enhanced tolerance to this stress. This line of reasoning, with the knowledge that cardiac ischemia causes stress protein induction [14,15], has prompted a number of investigators to examine whether tissue entering ischemia with a preelevation of stress proteins is resistant to infarction [16,17].

Stress protein properties and nomenclature

To understand the possible protective benefits of stress proteins, a brief description of their function is necessary. *Constitutive* stress proteins are expressed in the basal, unstressed state but will, by definition, be synthesized at higher levels during stress. Alternatively, stress proteins may be exclusively *inducible*, being present only in the stressed organism.

Stress proteins are grouped into families with differing functions [7,8,18], and their nomenclature is such that they are classified primarily according to molecular weight (Table 1).

Specifically, the stress protein families include those in the range 100–200, 80–100, 70, 58–65, and 25–30 kD and ubiquitin. In terms of function, hsp104 is thought to be essential in some organisms in confering thermotolerance [11]. Hsp104 and hsp70 perform similar functions in that they act as

Table 1. Summary of the main families of stress proteins

Family	Function of Family
100–200 kD	Chaparones functionally similar to HSP 70 family. e.g., HSP 104 confers thermotolerance [11]
80–100 kD	Bind to specific proteins to silence function or escort to correct cellular compartment. e.g., facilitates transport and prevents activation of steroid receptor [21]
70 kD	Dissociate protein aggregates. Maintain polypeptides in unfolded state and accelerate proper folding. *The major inducible stress protein within the heart. The most commonly used marker of the cardiac stress response.* e.g., Promote mitochondrial protein folding [23]; confers thermotolerance [12]
60 kD	Allow reassembly of complex proteins within the mitochondrion. e.g., Assembly of mitochondrial F1ATPase [27]
25–30 kD	Various members, some with antioxidant properties and others structural. e.g., αB-crystallin alters properties of actin [28]
Ubiquitin	Targets proteins destined for degradation [7]

molecular chaperones and are apparently partly interchangeable with a high degree of functional overlap between the two.

The 90-kD family bind actin, a phenomenon that is modulated by both calcium and calmodulin [19]. Their location is predominantly cytoplasmic, and they are thought to act as chaperones [20], being able to assist the transport of molecules through their interaction with actin filaments whilst also offering protection against inappropriate or premature molecular interactions. For example the 90-kD heat stress protein (hsp90) associates with the receptors for several different steroid hormones. This association anchors the receptors to actin filaments and prevents their premature activation. The binding of the appropriate hormone then results in dissociation of the receptor from hsp90 [21].

The 70-kD family bind and hydrolyze ATP [22], their release from polypeptide chains being an energy-dependent process. Amongst other functions, they are involved in post-translational import of proteins into endoplasmic reticula and mitochondria [23] and constitute the clathrin-uncoating ATPase, which dissociates clathrin triskelions from clathrin-coated vesicles during endocytosis [24]. One member of this family, the 72-kD stress protein, is highly inducible and the most frequently used marker of the cardiac stress response.

The 60-kD family of proteins is predominantly mitochondrial and is essential for facilitating the refolding of proteins imported from the cytoplasm. Nuclear encoded mitochondrial proteins are translocated via specific contact sites between the outer and inner mitochondrial membranes before proteolytic processing and interaction with mitochondrial hsp70 (mhsp70) and hsp60 in the matrix [23,25]. Hsp60 is associated with many components of the inner mitochondrial membrane, such as cytochrome reductase [26] and components of the assembled F1-ATPase complex [27].

Numerous other lower molecular weight stress proteins exist, the most highly conserved being ubiquitin, which, by binding to proteins, targets them for degradation [7]. The low molecular weight stress proteins in the range 20–30 kD, such as hsp27, share homology with the eye lens protein alpha-crystallin, which is associated with the cytoskeleton and alters the physical properties of actin and desmin [28]. The binding of alpha-crystallin to actin and desmin is increased at acidic pH and also following heat shock. The association of alpha-crystallin with these cytoskeletal proteins decreases their propensity to form aggregates at acidic pH, leading to the suggestion that may play a role in preventing filament aggregation and irreversible structural damage during ischemia [28]. In the myocardium hsp27 is induced rapidly following both heat shock [29] and ischemia [30]. Another low molecular weight stress protein, the 32-kD protein, probably has direct or indirect antioxidant properties, since it is induced (at least in skin fibroblasts [31]) by heavy metals, ultraviolet light, and hydrogen peroxide, and glutathione may be its intracellular target.

Cells exposed to elevated temperature or to other denaturing stresses will have a high content of abnormally folded or denatured proteins. In this situation, the stress proteins would act by minimizing the potentially damaging interactions of the denatured protein with other correctly folded proteins, the activity of which must be maintained to ensure cellular survival. In keeping with this hypothesis is the appearance of abnormal proteins in cells with artificially depressed stress protein levels [32].

The major heat stress proteins exhibit a strong evolutionary conservation, with homologous proteins being found in all organisms studies, from bacteria to humans. This evolutionary conservation has led to the suggestion that the stress proteins play a vitally important role in cellular processes, their presence apparently being necessary for an organism to survive adverse environmental changes and to pass genetic information to progeny. The resultant homology between bacterial and human stress proteins gives rise to shared epitopes, which have been implicated in human autoimmunity and diabetes [33,34]. Although a considerable amount is known about these proteins and their protective effects in different cell types, their relation to a protective role in the heart is still in its infancy.

STRESS PROTEINS AND THE HEART

Stress proteins have been detected in the myocardium of a variety of mammalian species. Their synthesis has been shown to be increased by whole-body temperature elevation [17,35–37] and other stressful stimuli, including ischemia [14], brief ischemia and reperfusion [15], anoxia [38], hypoxia [39], pressure or volume overload [40], mechanical stretch [41], and drugs such as vasopressin [42], isoproterenol [43], hydrogen peroxide [44], L-type (slow) calcium-channel blockers [45], and other cardiotoxic drugs and heavy metals [38,46]. The implication of these findings is that stress proteins may play an important role in the cardiac stress response. Although many of these stimuli induce members of the 70-kD family of stress proteins, there appear to be differences in the pattern of stress protein induction when other families of stress proteins are considered. For example, cardiotoxic drugs preferentially induce a 30-kD stress protein [46]. It is possible that each stress induces its own subtly different profile of stress proteins best suited to meet the cellular consequences of that particular stress.

In our laboratory it has been found that the pattern of expression of 60-kD and 70-kD stress proteins differ in response to ischemia and reperfusion; that is, ischemia results in preferential expression of hsp60, while reperfusion results in expression of hsp70 [47]. This suggests that individual stress protein genes may have different regulatory mechanisms. Taking this further, the individual biochemical components of a particular stress may have differing effects on different stress genes. Therefore, whether two different stimuli induce a similar pattern of gene expression may depend on whether they share similar biochemical characteristics. For instance, to what extent are heat stress and ischemia similar in terms of the stress protein response that they produce?

Heat stress and ethanol are known to produce crosstolerance, as defined previously. Although they are, at first sight, widely differing stresses, it is thought that thermotolerance is mediated largely via hsp70 induction. Both heat stress and ethanol treatment produce large amounts of denatured proteins, which are thought to be a major stimulus for hsp70 induction [48]. Therefore, it is the nature of the biochemical *lesion* produced that is important in determining the pattern of the stress response. Another major stimulus for hsp70 production in the myocardium appears to be oxygen-derived free radical production [49]. Differential sensitivity to various components of stress, such as free radical injury, may explain why, in our experience [47], hsp70 mRNA expression continues apace during reperfusion whilst hsp60 mRNA expression is only maintained during ischemia (Figure 1).

It would seem logical to predict that the expression of hsp60 mRNA during ischemia may be linked to mitochondrial lesions, such as damage to components of the respiratory chain. It has also been reported recently that some "stress" genes such as hsp70 and protein tyrosine phosphatases may be directly responsive to free radicals [50]. The response of tyrosine phosphatase genes to free radical stress gives an insight into the involvement of intracellular signalling mechanisms in mediating the stress response. This necessitates a broader conceptual understanding of the stress response to take into account factors other than stress proteins. With this in mind it is important to determine the biochemical nature of the molecular and cellular lesions produced by a particular stress (such as ischemia) and the resultant patterns of gene expression in order to properly design strategies that may harness

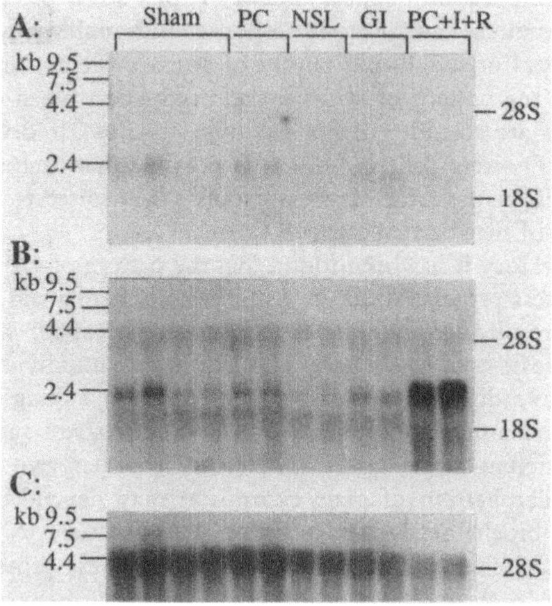

Figure 1. Northern blots demonstrating changes in mRNA for Hsp 60 and Hsp 70 following brief periods of ischemia. Total RNA was isolated and Northern blotting carried out using standard protocols. LV ischemic zone samples were taken from four sham-ligated hearts (sham); two preconditioned hearts (PC); two control non-sham-ligated hearts (NSL); two hearts subjected to 15 minutes ex vivo global ischemia (GI); two hearts subjected to preconditioning and subsequent ischemia/reperfusion (PC+I+R). Blots were probed for **A**. hsp60 transcripts using a cDNA probe encoding the C-terminal 60% of human hsp60; **B** hsp70 transcripts using a cDNA probe specific for all members (constitutive and inducible); **C**: 28S rRNA. Filters were sequentially stripped and reprobed in the above order. RNA size markers are shown on the left for comparison and positions of 28S and 18S rRNA on the right. Hsp60 probe (λ22a) hybridized to single band at approximately 2.4 kb. Hsp70 probe (DP8) hybridized to two bands at approximately 2.4 and 2.6 kb. **A**: PC (5 minutes ischemia + 10 minutes reperfusion) and GI (15 minutes global ischemia) showed a twofold increase in hsp60 transcript compared to 3 of the 4 sham-ligated and 2 of the 2 non-sham-ligated control hearts. Hsp60 mRNA returned to baseline following a subsequent 30-minute ischemia + 2 hours reperfusion (PC+I+R). **B**: An approximate twofold increase in hsp70 2.4-kb transcript was also evident following PC and GI. However, an additional 2.6-kb transcript that appeared during the subsequent 30-minute ischemic insult (not shown), accumulated to approximately 20 to 30-fold during the 2-hour reperfusion phase (PC+I+R). **C**: Analysis of the 28S rRNA shows approximately equal total RNA loadings for each sample.

the cells' own defenses. Such observations, in light of the phenomenon of crosstolerance, have prompted investigators to examine whether cardiac tissue with *preelevated* stress protein exhibits an enhanced resistance to a range of cardiac stresses.

HEAT STRESS AND MYOCARDIAL PROTECTION

Isolated heart and global ischemia

Currie et al. [16] were the first investigators to show that temperature elevation in rats to 42°C resulted in concomittant cardiac stress protein and catalase induction, and an attentuation of ischemia/reperfusion injury. Using an isolated heart model, these investigators demonstrated that following ischemia/reperfusion, contractile function is enhanced, whilst creatine kinase release is dramatically reduced in heat-stressed compared with control hearts. These findings have been confirmed by us in both the rat [51] as well as the rabbit [17]. Moreover, we have also observed an improvement in additional parameters of protection in the heat-stressed rabbit heart postischemia. These include preservation of high energy phosphates, a reduction in oxidative stress during reperfusion (as measured by lower levels of oxidized glutathione), and significant mitochondrial preservation following ischemia [17]. The ability of heat stress to enhance mitochondrial function is also supported by the observation that addition of pyruvate (a substrate that is readily oxidized) seems to enhance contractile performance following hypoxia and reoxygenation in heat-stressed papillary muscle [52]. There does, however, appear to be some species variation in the metabolic changes associated with protection following heat stress. In the rabbit, for example, we have demonstrated higher levels of high energy phosphates that mirror the enhanced contractile activity of heat-stressed hearts during reperfusion [17] (Figure 2). In the rat, however, the enhanced contractile activity following ischemia in the heat-stressed groups is not associated with differences in high-energy phosphate content between heat-stressed and control hearts [51,53].

Not all studies, however, have found heat stress to be cardioprotective. For example, preliminary studies by one group [54] have been unable to demonstrate any protection against "no-flow" ischemia following heat stress in the isolated unpaced working rat heart with rate-pressure product and cardiac output as end points. These investigators, although following an established protocol known to enhance cardiac stress protein synthesis, did not measure stress proteins directly.

Isolated heart and regional ischemia

The studies summarized to this point have demonstrated protection expressed in terms of myocardial contractility and metabolic state. The ability of whole-body heat stress to reduce the extent of myocardial infarction as examined by triphenyl tetrazolium staining has also been examined. In a preliminary study in the rat model infarct size is reduced following 37.5 minutes of regional ischemia, with protection being temporally related to elevated stress protein levels at 24–96 hours following whole-body heat stress [55]. In addition, we have demonstrated a similar reduction in infarct size following 45 minutes of regional ischemia and 2 hours reperfusion in the

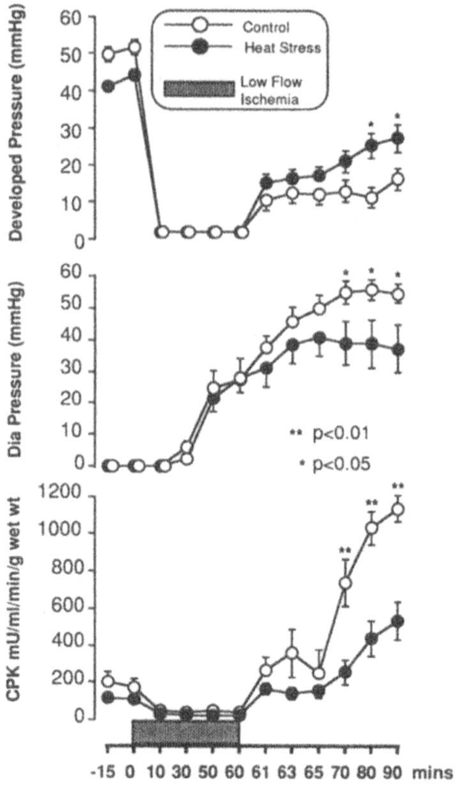

Figure 2. Left ventricular developed (top), end-diastolic (middle) pressure, and CPK release (bottom) in Langendorff-perfused rabbit hearts following 60 minutes of low-flow global ischemia. Heat stress was achieved by warming rabbits to 42°C for 15 minutes, and controls received anesthetic alone. Rabbits were allowed to recover for 24 hours prior to removal of hearts. Left ventricular developed pressure is significantly better preserved following reperfusion in heat-stressed hearts. Contracture assesed by left ventricular diastolic pressure is similar in heat stress and control hearts during ischaemia but less severe in the heat stress group during reperfusion. Similarly, CPK release on reperfusion is significantly less in heat stress hearts.

buffer perfused rabbit heart removed 24 hours after whole-body heat stress [56,57]. In this model heat stress reduced infarct size as a percentage of the myocardium at risk from 70.7 ± 4.4 in control hearts to 51.5 ± 5.7.

In situ heart and regional ischemia

Interestingly, in contrast to isolated heart studies, controversy surrounds the ability of whole-body heat stress to reduce infarct size in vivo. In the rabbit heat stress 24 hours prior to ischemia was unable to reduce infarct size following a 45-minute coronary occlusion [58], although an effect was apparent with a 30-minute occlusion [59]. A similar dependence on the length of coronary occlusion is seen in the rat. Donnelly and coworkers have demonstrated a reduction in infarct size in the rat following a 35-minute, but not a 45-minute, coronary occlusion initiated 24 hours after whole-body heat stress [60]. The apparent dependency of protection on the length of ischemic insult is difficult to explain. One possibility is that the protection conferred by heat stress is only moderate, and that as the severity of the ischemic insult increases the protection becomes less evident. A similar phenomenon occurs with ischemic preconditioning in dogs, in which a marked reduction in infarct size occurs with 60 minutes of coronary occlusion, but not with 90 minutes [61].

Other investigators have also been able to demonstrate in vivo protection following hot blood cardioplegia of the pig heart [62]. In another rather novel approach [63], a microwave diathermy probe was applied to the canine heart. Although such regional hyperthermia was shown to increase stress protein mRNA expression, there was no concomitant protection against infarction. However, the time course of this study was such that appreciable stress protein accumulation was unlikely to have occurred in the 1 hour between thermal stress and coronary ligation. In addition, the spatial relationship between heat-treated myocardium and the subsequent area of hypoperfusion during coronary ligation was unclear [63].

The cause for the discrepancy between in vivo and in vitro studies is unclear. However, recent observations from our laboratory suggest that whole-body heat stress may activate a blood borne component that overrides the beneficial effect of cardiac stress protein induction. This inference was made after we noticed that blood from a heat-stressed support rabbit, when used to perfuse an isolated rabbit heart, significantly increased infarct size [57]. It may be that whole-body heat stress, although conferring myocardial protection, causes confounding physiological changes that have negative effects on infarct size. In addition, the duration of recovery after heat stress and the length of the ischemic insult also appear to influence the cardioprotective effects.

HEAT STRESS PROTEINS AND CLASSICAL ISCHEMIC PRECONDITIONING

Acquired thermotolerance, where sublethal temperature elevation protects against subsequent lethal hyperthermia, is similar in concept to ischemic preconditioning, with sublethal ischemia protecting against subsequent lethal ischemia. However, the time course of acquired protection is different in each case. One could speculate that stress proteins synthesized in response to the first brief episode of preconditioning ischemia are involved in the protection against the subsequent injury. In agreement with this idea, Knowlton et al. [15] demonstrated that brief bursts of ischemia, such as those used in preconditioning protocols, can induce hsp70 mRNA and protein accumulation. The mechanism by which stress proteins are induced by short episodes of ischemia may be secondary to the free radical stress induced by reperfusion, since in the isolated rat heart stress protein induction following a 15-minute infusion of xanthine plus xanthine oxidase is quantitatively similar to that induced by ischemia with reperfusion [49]. However, in both the Knowlton study [15] and our own work [64], elevated levels of the hsp70 protein were only manifest at 2–24 hours after the ischemic insult. In contrast the protective effect of preconditioning is lost approximately 1 hour after the initial brief ischemic episode [65].

The involvement of stress protein in ischemic preconditioning has been further questioned by a study [67] that indicates the protective effect of preconditioning can be observed under conditions in which de novo protein synthesis has been almost entirely inhibited. It should be noted, however, that the efficacy of the inhibitors was only measured with respect to total protein synthesis. The possibility that one or more stress proteins continue to be made under these conditions cannot be excluded [46]. Furthermore, all the work examining the relationship between stress proteins and ischemic preconditioning performed to date has focused on the 70-kD heat stress protein, ignoring other families of stress proteins. However, initial studies in our own laboratory have shown changes at the mRNA level of the 60-kD mitochondrial stress protein (hsp60) within minutes of the onset of ischemia (Figure 1) [67]. The rapid increase in the levels of hsp60 mRNA was closely coupled to the presence of ischemia and apparently not dependent on components of reperfusion, in contrast to hsp70 mRNA as described above. Furthermore, the induction of hsp60 transcripts may be coupled to adenosine release during ischemia, since preliminary results from our laboratory indicate that this induction may be blocked by the nonspecific adenosine receptor antagonist 8-sulphophenyl theophylline (8-SPT). Hsp70 mRNA production was not affected by 8-SPT, again emphasizing that hsp60 and hsp70 genes may be regulated by different mechanisms and different biochemical components of the same stress. Despite this rapid increase in hsp60 mRNA levels, no change in hsp60 or hsp70 protein was detected by Western blot analysis over the time course of preconditioning. Thus, it remains unlikely that stress proteins are involved in *classical ischemic preconditioning*. However, the changes in mRNA coding for stress proteins indicate an adaptive response to ischemia that may predict a *delayed protection dependent on stress protein synthesis*.

A further difficulty in attempting to dissociate ischemic preconditioning from stress protein synthesis is that post-transcriptional mechanisms such as translocation of stress protein within the cell may have an equally important functional role as alterations in total cellular content [68]. Such intracellular translocations occur rapidly during anoxia and may not be influenced by protein synthesis inhibition. However, until other families of stress proteins and stress protein translocations are examined in more detail, their involvement, or otherwise, in this acute protective phenomenon cannot be categorically ruled out.

NONTHERMALLY INDUCED STRESS PROTEINS AND PROTECTION AGAINST ISCHEMIA

The fact that stress protein induction by ischemia is not temporally related to classical ischemic preconditioning has prompted some of us to examine whether preconditioning ischemia is associated with a delayed, as well as an early phase of myocardial protection. Preliminary reports using the dog model [69,70] suggest that a second phase of protection exists at 24 hours after preconditioning with four repeated 5-minute episodes of ischemia. We have also found a similar reduction in infarct size in the rabbit at 24 hours after a similar preconditioning regimen [59] and have demonstrated that the content of myocardial hsp72 within the risk zone is equivalent to that seen within the left ventricle following whole-body heat stress (Figures 3 and 4). However, in a preliminary study using a similar protocol but without stress

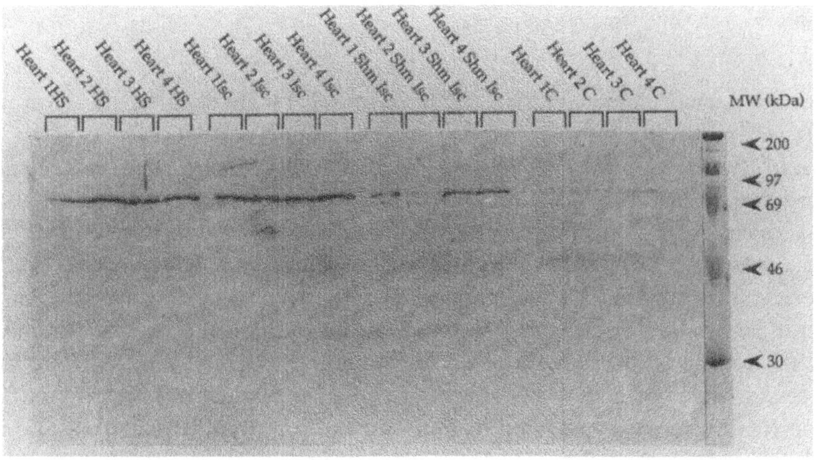

Figure 3. Western blot immunoprobed with a monoclonal IgG against the inducible 70-kD stress protein. Samples were derived from left ventricular tissue from four experimental groups, each comprising four hearts. Hearts 1HS to 4HS (heat stress group) were from rabbits warmed to 42°C for 15 minutes. Hearts 1Isc to 4Isc were rendered ischemic in situ by four periods of 5 minutes of coronary ligation, each separated by 10 minutes of reperfusion. Hearts 1Shm Isc to 4Shm Isc were from rabbits that underwent median sternotomy and pericardiotomy without regional ischemia, and hearts 1C to 4C were from rabbits that received anesthetic agent alone and acted as a control for the heat stress group. All rabbits were allowed to recover for 24 hours before hearts were removed for stress protein analysis. Protein loading is approximately equal for all groups. The inducible 70-kD stress protein is seen to migrate with the trailing edge of the 69-kD molecular weight marker. On the basis of densitometric assessment, induction in heat stress and ischemia pretreatment groups is similar and significantly greater than in corresponding controls.

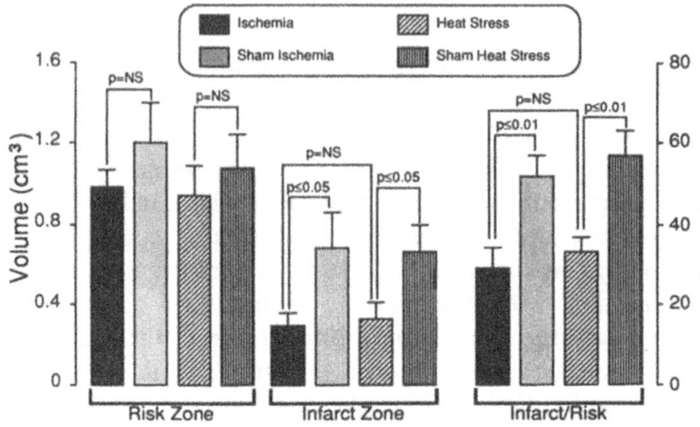

Figure 4. Infarct sizes following 30 minutes of regional ischemia and 2 hours of reperfusion in each of the four groups described in the legend for Figure 3. Comparisons are by ANOVA. Both heat stress and ischemic pretreatments are associated with a significant reduction in both absolute infarct volume and infarct volume expressed as a percentage of the volume of tissue at risk. Infarct volume was determined using triphenyltetrazolium staining, and area at risk was delineated with flourescent microspheres.

protein measurements, other investigators [71] have failed to demonstrate delayed protection. Interestingly, a similar phenomenon appears to occur within the brain, where ischemic pretreatment with two repeated episodes of 2-minute bilateral carotid occlusions is capable of limiting the neuronal cell loss that follows a subsequent more prolonged bilateral carotid occlusion [72]. For this protective effect to be manifest, the short occlusions must precede the long occlusion by at least 24 hours, a time interval known to result in cerebral heat stress protein induction in an identical model [73]. Other methods of stress protein induction have included immobilization stress, which has also been shown to protect against subsequent ischemia/reperfusion injury as assessed by CK leakage, contractile function, and reperfusion arrhythmias [74,75]. It is interesting to speculate that myocardial adaptation to ischemia may explain the apparent benefit of a 7-day or more history of angina prior to myocardial infarction [76], although likely collateral vessel formation, concomitant medication and contradictory findings [77] make any definite conclusions impossible.

In contrast other attempts to induce myocardial protection by ischemic pretreatment have been unsuccesful. For example, Donnelly et al. [60] compared the protective benefit of heat stress with 24 hours of recovery to 20 minutes of ischemia with 8 hours of reperfusion. Following a subsequent 35-minute occlusion in the rat, heat stress pretreatment reduced infarct size whilst ischemic pretreatment did not. However, as heat stress resulted in a more marked stress protein accumulation, the authors concluded that protection was absent following ischemic pretreatment because of insufficient stress protein accumulation.

PROTECTION AGAINST NONISCHEMIC INJURY

The observations that cardiac tissues synthesize stress proteins in response to a variety of stresses has encouraged investigators to explore the breadth of protection that follows heat stress. In this regard Meerson [78,79], as well as ourselves [80], have demonstrated that stress protein induction by either heat or immobilization protects the isolated rat and rabbit heart against a subsequent calcium paradox. The interesting aspect of this finding is that, unlike ischemia/reperfusion injury, reactive oxygen species are not involved in the genesis of the calcium paradox. This implies that myocardial protection associated with stress protein induction is not dependent upon antioxidant mechanisms.

The fact that oxidant stress is capable of inducing cardiac stress proteins [44,48] has prompted Su et al. [81] to examine the protective benefits of prior heat stress with exposure to H_2O_2 as the final stress. In a rat myocyte culture model, heat stress is capable of inducing acquired thermotolerance and limiting myocyte injury on subsequent H_2O_2 exposure. More importantly, transfecting the same culture system so as to overexpress the human inducible hsp70 (hsp72) causes cells to become more tolerant to simulated ischemia [82]. This provides the most direct evidence to date that stress proteins per se, rather than the nonspecific effects of heat stress, are responsible for myocardial protection. A further indication that stress proteins may be direct mediators of myocardial protection is the observation that, in rabbit papillary muscle, contractile recovery following hypoxia/reoxygenation is correlated with the stress protein content of adjacent myocardial tissue [83].

MECHANISMS OF CARDIAC PROTECTION BY ELEVATED TEMPERATURE

All studies using heat to elevate stress protein synthesis result in a large number of physiological perturbations [84], which may in themselves have cardioprotective properties. For example, Currie's group [16,85] have shown that heat stress also results in an increase in the endogenous levels of the antioxidant enzyme catalase. Moreover, they have demonstrated [84] that inactivating catalase with 3-AT (3-aminotriazole) results in an abolition of the protective effect normally observed at 24 and 48 hours after heat stress. This protective role of catalase would be dependent upon its ability to minimize the damage caused by secondary free radical generation to sulfhydryl-containing enzymes, DNA, and lipids [86] by catalyzing the conversion of H_2O_2 to water. Following a period of prolonged ischemia, the importance of catalase is increased, since there is a marked reduction in the activity of SOD as well as in the ratio of reduced to oxidized glutathione [86]. In agreement with such a mechanism, we have observed a reduction in the levels of oxidized glutathione in the coronary effluent following ischemia/reperfusion in heat-stressed hearts, suggesting that a second, alternative line of antioxidant defense exists in these hearts [17]. The picture, however, becomes more complicated, since cardiac mRNA levels for catalase are not increased by heat stress [29]. The increase in catalase may therefore result from post-translational mechanisms. An alternative suggestion is that stress proteins may modulate the activity of catalase by direct interaction with the enzyme [87].

As mentioned previously, other evidence suggests that stress proteins may be able to limit myocardial damage independent of an antioxidant effect. Two recent reports suggest that the injury occurring during the calcium paradox can be influenced by procedures that cause stress protein synthesis [78,80]. The precise mode by which the calcium paradox damages the heart is a matter of controversy, but free-radical production is probably not involved [88]. It is thought that during the period of low calcium exposure changes occur in the structural proteins of the myocyte so as to increase fragility, and, on calcium repletion, the return of contractile activity causes myocyte mechanical disruption [89]. A similar process involving cytoskeletal disruption may also occur during ischemia [90]. Heat stress proteins are known to alter the physical properties of actin and desmin [28], and may themselves form an integral part of the cytoskeleton [91]. As already mentioned it has been postulated that they may attenuate ischemia/reperfusion injury by binding to and stabilizing the cytoskeleton during ischemia [28].

Yet another possible mechanism of protection is that during heat stress, protein synthesis (apart from the stress proteins) is inhibited. A similar response has been noted during other forms of stress in cardiac tissue [92], and it has been postulated that such a response allows the cell to redirect energy into more vital cell processes during and following times of stress. A 17-kD stress protein that inhibits protein translation has been isolated from cardiac tissue and is expressed in response to heat and pressure overload [93], providing yet another possible mechanism by which heat stress confers myocardial protection.

FUTURE DIRECTIONS

A number of potential mechanisms exist by which the heart might be protected following heat stress. In order to elucidate whether stress proteins are the true mediators of this protection, it will be necessary to individually overexpress each of the stress proteins in cardiac cells either in culture or in transgenic animals. By measuring whether such cells are protected from various stresses, such as ischemia, it will be possible to assess which stress proteins mediate the protection against which stress.

CONCLUSIONS

The cross-species conservation of stress proteins suggest they play a vital role in preserving cell viability, a hypothesis that has been confirmed by the fact that their manipulation can alter cellular vulnerability to stress. Stress proteins are induced in the heart by various physiological and pathological conditions, such as ischemia, implying that they may have a role in recovery from such stresses. These observations have prompted studies in which the stress protein content of the heart is elevated by heat stress prior to ischemia. The protective effect of elevated temperature on the ability of the heart to survive a subsequent stress has now been demonstrated by a number of different laboratories using different animal species with various end points.

Stress proteins are induced by the brief periods of sublethal ischemia known to cause ischemic preconditioning. However, since, the induction of the stress proteins so far tested does not correlate with the timing of classical ischemic preconditioning, they are unlikely to be involved in this phenomenon.

The weight of evidence presented suggests that stress proteins influence the resistance of the heart to ischemia and may offer an *endogenous route to myocardial protection*. Such a route represents an obvious pathway for therapeutic intervention. Further studies will be necessary to pave the way for the rational design and testing of therapeutic agents to augment stress protein synthesis. It is hoped that in the future it may be possible to protect the heart by a specific but nonabusive stimulation of its own protective mechanisms.

ACKNOWLEDGMENTS

We are grateful to the British Heart Foundation and the Hatter Foundation for their continued support. Michael S Marber is the recipient of a British Heart Foundation Intermediate Fellowship.

REFERENCES

1. Maroko PR, Kjekshus JK, Sobel BE, Watanabe T, Covell JW, Ross J, Braunwald E. 1971. Factors influencing infarct size following experimental coronary artery occlusion. Circulation 43:67–82.
2. Hearse DJ, Yellon DM. 1984. Why are we still in doubt about infarct size limitation? The experimentalists viewpoint. In Therepeutic Approaches to Myocardial Infarct Size Limitation. DJ Hearse, DM Yellon, eds. Raven Press, New York, pp. 17–41.
3. Chambers DE, Yellon DM, Hearse DJ, Downey JM. 1983. Effects of flurbiprofen in altering the size of myocardial infarcts in dogs: Reduction or delay? Am J Cardiol 51:884–890.
4. Hearse DJ, Yellon DM, Downey JM. 1986. Can beta blockers limit infarct size? Eur Heart J 7:925–930.
5. Murry CE, Jennings RB, Reimer KA. 1986. Preconditioning with ischemia: A delay of lethal cell injury in ischemic myocardium. Circulation 74:1124–1136.
6. Yellon DM, Latchman DS. 1992. Stress proteins and myocardial protection. J Mol Cell Cardiol 24:113–124.
7. Lindquist S. 1986. The heat shock response. Ann Rev Biochem 55:1151–1191.
8. Hightower LE. 1991. Heat shock, stress proteins, chaperones, and proteotoxicity. Cell 66:191–197.
9. Pelham HRB. 1986. Speculation on the functions of the major heat shock and glucose related proteins. Cell 46:959–961.
10. Bansal GS, Norton PM, Latchman DS. 1991. The 90kd heat shock protein protects cells from thermal stress but not from viral infection. Exp Cell Res 195:303–306.
11. Sanchez Y, Lindquist SL. 1990. HSP104 required for induced thermotolerance. Science 248:1112–1115.

12. Angelidis CE, Lazaridis I, Papoulatos GN. 1991. Constitutive expression of heat-shock protein 70 in mammalian cells confers thermoresistance. Eur J Biochem 199:35–39.
13. Li GC. 1983. Induction of thermotolerance and enhanced heat shock protein synthesis in Chinese hamster fibroblasts by sodium arsenite and by ethanol. J Cell Physiol 115:116–122.
14. Mehta HB, Popovich BK, Dillman WH. 1988. Ischemia induces changes in the level of mRNAs coding for stress protein 71 and creatine kinase M. Circ Res 63:512–517.
15. Knowlton AA, Brecher P, Apstein CS. 1990. Rapid expression of heat shock protein in the rabbit after brief cardiac ischemia. J Clin Invest 87:139–147.
16. Currie RW, Karmazyn M, Kloc M, Mailer K. 1988. Heat shock response is associated with enhanced postischemic ventricular recovery. Circ Res 63:543–549.
17. Yellon DM, Pasini E, Cargnoni A, Marber MS, Latchman DS, Ferrari R. 1992. The protective role of heat stress in the ischaemic and reperfused rabbit myocardium. J Mol Cell Cardiol 24:895–907.
18. Welch WJ. 1990. The mammalian stress response: Cell physiology and biochemistry of stress proteins. In Stress Proteins in Biology and Medicine. R Morimoto, A Tissieres, C Georgopoulos, eds. Cold Spring Laboratory Press, Cold Spring Harbor, NY, pp. 223–229.
19. Koyasu S, Nishida E, Miyata Y, Sakai H, Yahara I. 1989. HSP 100, a 100-kDa heat shock protein, is a Ca^{2+}-calmodulin-regulated actin binding protein. J Biol Chem 264: 15083–15087.
20. Ellis RJ. 1990. Molecular chaperones. Semin Cell Biol 1:1–72.
21. Miyata Y, Yahara I. 1991. Cytoplasmic 8S glucocorticoid receptor binds to actin filaments through the 90-kDa heat shock protein moiety. J Biol Chem 266:8779–8783.
22. Flaherty KM, DeLuca-Flaherty C, McKay DB. 1990. Three-dimensional structure of the ATPase fragment of a 70K heat-shock cognate protein. Nature 346:623–628.
23. Kang P, Ostermann J, Shilling J, Neupert W, Craig EA, Pfanner N. 1990. Requirement for HSP70 in the mitochondrial matrix for translocation and folding of precursor proteins. Nature 348:137–143.
24. Chappell TG, Welch WJ, Schlossman DM, Palter KB, Schlessinger MJ, Rothman JE. 1986. Uncoating ATPase is a member of the 70 kDa family of stress proteins Cell 45:3–12.
25. Horwich A. 1990. Protein import into mitochondria and peroxisomes. Current Opin Cell Biol 2:625–633.
26. Hutchinson EG, Tichelaar W, Hofhaus G, Weiss H, Leonard KR. 1989. Identification and electron microscopic analysis of a chaperonin oligomer from *Nuerospora crassa* mitochondria. EMBO J 8:1485–1490.
27. Gray RE, Grasso DG, Maxwell RJ, Finnegan PM, Nagley P, Devennish RJ. 1990. Identification of 66 kDa protein associated with yeast mitochondrial ATP synthase as heat shock protein hsp60. FEBS Let 268:265–268.
28. Bennardini F, Wrzosek A, Chiesi M. 1992. αB-crystallin in cardiac tissue. Association with actin and desmin filaments. Circ Res 71:288–294.
29. Currie RW, Tanguay RM. 1991. Analysis of RNA for transcripts for catalase and SP71 in rat hearts after in vivo hyperthermia. Biochem Cell Biol 69:375–382.
30. Andres J, Sharma HS, Knoll R, Sassen L, Verdouw PD. 1992. Enhanced expression of mRNAs encoding ubiquitin and hsp27 in porcine stunned myocardium. Circulation 86(Suppl I):I624 (abstr).
31. Keyse SM, Tyrell RM. 1982. Both near ultra violet radiation and the oxidising agent hydrogen peroxide induce a 32 kDa stress protein in normal human skin fibroblasts. J Biol Chem 262:14821–14825.
32. Dorner AJ, Krane MG, Kaufman RJ. 1988. Reduction of endogenous GRP78 levels in CHO cells and its effects on secretion. J Cell Biochem 12D(Suppl):276 (abstr).
33. Harboe M, Quayla AJ. 1991. Heart shock proteins: Friend and foe? Clin Exp Immounol 21:2–5.
34. Latchman DS. 1991. Heat shock proteins and human disease. J R Coll Physicians Lond 25:295–299.
35. Currie RW, White FP. 1983. Characterization of the synthesis and accumulation of a 71-kilodalton protein induced in rat tissues after hyperthermia. Can J Biochem Cell Biol 61:438–446.
36. Currie RW. 1987. Effects of ischemia and perfusion temperature on the synthesis of stress induced (heat shock) proteins in isolated and perfused rat hearts. J Mol Cell Cardiol 19:795–808.

37. Iwaki K, Mestril R, Dillman WH, Chien KR. 1989. Induction of HSP 71 mRNA correlates with arachidonic acid release and the transition to irreversible injury in neonatal rat myocardial cells following ATP depletion. Circulation 80(Suppl II):II462 (abstr).
38. Tuijl MJ, van Bergen en Henegouwen PM, van Wijk R, Verkleij AJ. 1991. The isolated neonatal rat-cardiomyocyte used as an in vitro model for "ischemia." II. Induction of the 68 kDa heat shock protein. Biochim Biophys Acta 1091:278–284.
39. Howard G, Geoghegan TE. 1986. Altered cardiac tissue gene expression during acute hypoxic exposure. Mol Cell Biochem 69:155–160.
40. Delcayre C, Samuel JL, Marrothe F, Mescadier JJ, Rappaport L. 1988. Synthesis of stress proteins in rat cardiac myocytes 2–4 days after imposition of hemodynamic overload. J Clin Invest 82:460–468.
41. Knowlton AA, Eberli FR, Brecher P, Romo GM, Owen A, Apstein CS. 1991. A single myocardial stretch or decreased systolic fiber shortening stimulates the expression of heat shock protein 70 in the isolated, erythrocyte-perfused rabbit heart. J Clin Invest 88:2018–2025.
42. Moalic JM, Bauters C, Himbert D, Bercovici J, Mouas C, Guicheney P, Baudoin-Legras M, Rappaport L, Emanoil-Ravier R, Mezger V, Swynghedauw B. 1989. Phenylepinephrine, vasopressin and angiotensin as determinants of heat shock protein gene expression in adult rat heart and aorta. J Hypertens 7:195–201.
43. White FP, White SC. 1986. Isoproterenol induced myocardial necrosis is associated with stress protein synthesis in rat heart and thoracic aorta. Cardiovasc Res 20:512–515.
44. Low I, Friedrich T, Schoeppe W. 1989. Synthesis of shock proteins in cultured fetal mouse myocardial cells. Exp Cell Res 180:451–459.
45. Löw-Friedrich I, Schoeppe W. 1991. Effects of calcium channel blockers on stress protein synthesis in cardiac myocytes. J Cardiovasc Pharmacol 17:800–806.
46. Löw-Friedrich I, von Bredow F, Schoeppe W. 1991. A cell culture system for the detection of cardiotoxicity. J Pharmacol Methods 25:133–145.
47. Heads RJ, Patel VC, Latchman DS, Yellon DM. 1992. Different expression patterns for 65kDa and 70kDa stress proteins following ischemic preconditioning. Circulation 86(Suppl I):I556 (abstr).
48. Ananthan J, Goldberg AL, Voellmy R. 1986. Abnormal proteins serve as eukaryotic stress signals and trigger the activation of heat shock genes. Science 232:252–254.
49. Kukreja RC, Batra SK, Loesser KE, Hess MLJ. 1992. Direct expression of heat shock protein by oxygen radicals in the isolated, perfused rat heart. J Mol Cell Cardiol 24(Suppl I):S101 (abstr).
50. Keyse SM, Emslie EA. 1992. Oxidative stress and heat shock induce a human gene encoding a protein-tyrosine phosphatase. Nature 359:644–647.
51. Pasini E, Cargnoni A, Ferrari R, Marber MS, Latchman DS, Yellon DM. 1991. Heat stress and oxidative damage following ischemia and reperfusion in the isolated rat heart. Eur Heart J 12(Suppl):306 (abstr).
52. Marber MS, Walker JM, Latchman DS, Yellon DM. 1991. The resistance of rabbit papillary muscle to high flow anoxia is enhanced by heat stress when pyruvate is used as substrate. Circulation 84(Suppl II):II621 (abstr).
53. Currie RW, Karmazyn M. 1990. Improved post-ischemic ventricular recovery in the absence of changes in energy metabolism in working rat hearts following heat shock. J Mol Cell Cardiol 22:631–636.
54. Wall SR, Fliss H, Kako KJ, Korecky B. 1990. Heat pretreatment does not improve recovery of function after no-flow ischemia in isolated working rat hearts. J Mol Cell Cardiol (Suppl 1):S44 (abstr).
55. Loesser KE, Vinnikova AK, Qian YZ, Hess ML, Jesse RL, Kukreja RC. 1992. Protection of ischemia/reperfusion injury by heat stress in rats. Circulation 86(Suppl I):I557.
56. Walker DM, Kucukoglu S, Marber MS, Walker JM, Yellon DM. 1992. Heat stress limits infarct size in the isolated rabbit heart. Circulation 86(Suppl I):I557 (abstr).
57. Walker DM, Pasini E, Kucukoglu S, Marber MS, Iliodromitis E, Ferrari R, Yellon DM. 1993. Heat stress limits infarct size in the isolated perfused rabbit heart. Cardiovasc Res 27:962–967.
58. Yellon DM, Iliodromitis E, Latchman DS, Van Winkle DM, Downey JM, Williams FM, Williams TJ. 1992. Whole body heat shock fails to limit infarct size in the reperfused rabbit heart. Cardiovasc Res 26:342–346.

59. Marber MS, Latchman DS, Walker JM, Yellon DM. 1993. Cardiac stress protein elevation 24 hours following brief ischemia of heat stress is associated with resistance to myocardial infarction. Circulation 88:1264–1272.
60. Donnelly TJ, Sievers RE, Vissern FLJ, Welch WJ, Wolfe CL. 1992. Heat shock protein induction in rat hearts. A role for improved myocardial salvage after ischemia and reperfusion? Circulation 85:796–778.
61. Nao BS, McClanahan TB, Groh MA, Schott RJ, Gallagher KP. 1990. The time limit of effective ischemic preconditioning in dogs. Circulation 82(Suppl III):271 (abstr).
62. Liu X, Engelman RM, Moraru II, Rousou JA, Flack JE, Deaton DW, Maulik N, Das DK. 1992. Heat shock: A new approach for myocardial preservation in cardiac surgery. Circulation 86(Suppl II):II358–II363.
63. Schott R, Nao B, Strieter R, Groh M, Kunkel S, McClanahan T, Schaper W, Gallagher K. 1990. Heat shock does not precondition canine myocardium. Circulation 82(Suppl III):III464 (abstr).
64. Kucukogku S, Iliodromitis E, Van Winkle D, Downey J, Marber M, Heads R, Yellon DM. 1991. Protection by ischaemic preconditioning appears independent of stress protein synthesis. J Mol Cell Cardiol 23(Suppl V):S73 (abstr).
65. Van Winkle DM, Thorntom J, Downey JM. 1991. Cardioprotection from ischaemic preconditioning is lost following prolonged reperfusion in the rabbit. Coronary Artery Dis 2:613–619.
66. Thornton JD, Striplin S, Liu GS, Swafford A, Stanley WH, Van Winkle DM, Downety JM, 1990. Inhibition of protein synthesis does not block myocardial protection afforded by preconditioning. Am J Physiol 259:H1822–H1825.
67. Heads RJ, Patel VC, Latchman DS, Yellon DM. 1992. Ischaemic preconditioning causes rapid elevation of 65kD stress protein in rabbit heart. J Mol Cell Cardiol 24(Suppl I):S94 (abstr).
68. Snoeckx LHEH, Contard F, Samuel JL, Marotte F, Rappaport L. 1991. Expression and cellular distribution of heat-shock and nuclear oncogene proteins in rat hearts. Am J Physiol 261:LH1443–H1451.
69. Yamashita N, Kuzuya T, Hoshido S, Fuji H, Oe H, Kitabatake A, Tada M, Kamada T. 1992. Relationship between time interval from preconditioning to sustained ischemia and its effects on limiting infarct size. J Mol Cell Cardiol 24(Suppl I):S150 (abstr).
70. Hoshida S, Kuzuya T, Yamashita N, Fuji H, Oe H, Otsu K, Kimura Y, Hori M, Tada M. 1992. Delayed effect of sublethal ischemia on limiting infarct size resulting from sustained ischemia and reperfusion. Circulation: 86(Suppl I):I30 (abstr).
71. Tanaka M, Fujiwara H, Yamasaki K. ls the time course of infarct size limiting effect of ischemic preconditioning bimodal? Circulation 86(Suppl I):I343 (abstr).
72. Kitagawa K, Matsumoto M, Tagaya M, Hata R, Ueda H, Niinobe M, Handa N, Fukunaga R, Kimura K, Mikoshiba K, Kamada T. 1990. Ischemic tolerance phenomenon found in the brain. Brain Res 528:21–24.
73. Nowak TS. 1990. Protein synthesis and heat shock/stress response after ischemia. Cerebrovasc Brain Metab Rev 2:345–366.
74. Meerson FZ, Malyshev IY. 1989. Adaptation to stress increases the heart resistance to ischemic and reperfusion arrhythmias. J Mol Cell Cardiol 21:299–303.
75. Meerson FZ, Malyshew IY, Zamotrinsky AV. 1992. Differences in adaptive stabilization of structures in response to stress and hypoxia relate with the accumulation of hsp70 isoforms. Mol Cell Biochem III:87–95.
76. Muller DW, Topol EJ, Califf RM, Sigmon KN, Gorman L, George BS, Kereiakes DJ, Lee KL, Ellis SG. 1990. Relationship between antecedent angina pectoris and short-term prognosis after thrombolytic therapy for acute myocardial infarction. Thrombolysis and angioplasty in myocardial infarction (TAMI) study group. Am Heart J 119:224–231.
77. Behar S, Reicher-Reiss H, Allmader E. 1992. The prognostic significance of angina pectoris preceeding the occurrence of a first acute myocardial infarction in 4166 consecutive hospitalized patients. Am Heart J 123:1481–1486.
78. Meerson FZ, Malyshev IU, Arkhipenko YV, Vovk VI. 1991. Adaptive increase in the resistance of the heart to calcium paradox. J Mol Cell Cardiol 23(Suppl V):S162 (abstr).
79. Meerson FZ, Malyshev Y, Shneider AB. 1991. Phenomenon of the adaptive stabilization of sarcoplasmic and nuclear structures in myocardium. In Current Topics in Heart Failure. Steinkopff Verlag, Dermstadt.

80. Marber MS, Walker JM, Yellon DM. 1992. Heat stress can protect the rabbit heart by antioxidant independent mechanisms. Circulation 84(Suppl I):I556 (abstr).
81. Su C-Y, Dillmann WH, Woods WT, Owen OE. 1992. Heat shock induced oxidative tolerance in muscle cells. Circulation 84(Suppl I):I33 (abstr).
82. Mestril R, Chi S-H, Sayen RM, Dillmann WH. 1992. Expression of a human heat shock protein in rat heart derived H9c2 cells confers resistance against ischemic injury. Circulation 86(Suppl I):I557 (abstr).
83. Marber MS, Walker JM, Latchman DS, Yellon DM. 1992. Myocardial resistance to hypoxia is related to the content of the 72kDa stress protein. Circulation 86:I557 (abstr).
84. Gisolfi CV, Matthes RD, Kregel KC, Oppliger R. 1991. Splanchnic sympathetic nerve activity and circulating catecholamines in the hyperthermic rat. J Appl Physiol 70:1821–1826.
85. Karmazyn M, Mailer K, Currie RW. 1991. Acquisition and decay of heat shock enhanced post-ischemic ventricular recovery. Am J Physiol 259:H424–H431.
86. Ceconi C, Curello S, Cargnoni A, Ferrari R, Albertini A, Visioli O. 1988. The role of glutathione status in the protection against ischaemic and reperfusion damage: Effect of N-acetyl cysteine. J Mol Cell Cardiol 20:5–13.
87. Kukreja RC, Hess ML. 1992. The oxygen free radical system: From equations through membrane protein interactions to cardiovascular injury and protection. Cardiovasc Res 26:641–655.
88. Ferrari R, Ceconi C, Curello S, Cargnoni A, Ruigrok TJC. 1989. No evidence of oxygen free radical mediated damage during the calcium paradox. Basic Res Cardiol 84:396–403.
89. Altschuld RA, Ganote CE, Nayler WG, Piper HM. 1991. Editorial comment: What constitutes the calcium parardox? J Mol Cell Cardiol 23:765–767.
90. Steenbergen C, Hill ML, Jennings RB. 1987. Cytoskeletal damage during myocardial ischemia: Changes in Vinculin immunofluorescence staining during total in vitro ischemia in canine heart. Circ Res 60:478–486.
91. Green LA, Liem RK. 1989. Beta-internexin is a microtubule-associated protein identical to the heat-shock cognate protein and the clathrin uncoating ATPase. J Biol Chem 264: 15210–15215.
92. Havre PA, Hammond GL. 1988. Isolation of a translation-inhibiting peptide from myocardium. Am J Physiol 225:H1024–1031.
93. Hammond GL, Lai YK, Markert CL. 1992. Diverse forms of stress lead to new patterns of gene expression through a common and essential metabolic pathway. Proc Natl Acad Sci 79:3483–3488.

7. ROLE OF ATP-SENSITIVE POTASSIUM CHANNELS IN ISCHEMIC PRECONDITIONING

GARRETT J. GROSS, ZHENHAI YAO, and JOHN A. AUCHAMPACH

INTRODUCTION

In 1983, the ATP-sensitive potassium channel (K_{ATP}) was discovered in guinea pig ventricular myocytes by Noma [1] using the patch-clamp technique. In his original studies, Noma [1] found that the probability of this K channel being open was regulated primarily by intracellular concentrations of ATP in the micromolar range (25–200 μM) and, to a lesser extent, by ADP. These channels have been shown to exist in other tissues, such as the pancreas, CNS, and smooth muscle [2], where they have been postulated to be involved in insulin secretion, neurotransmitter release, and vascular smooth muscle relaxation, respectively. These channels are also found in skeletal muscle and kidney; however, their function in these tissues is still not clear. Subsequently, other important modulators of this channel have been identified, including pH, lactate, the ATP/ADP ratio, and the concentrations of other intracellular nucleotides [2,3]. In vivo, these other modulators of the channel appear to be as important in determining K_{ATP} channel opening as ATP concentrations, since the ATP level during early ischemia is in the millimolar (1–2 mM) range, whereas in in vitro patch clamp experiments ATP in the micromolar range regulate channel opening and closing [3].

Since the K_{ATP} channel is rapidly opened during ischemia or hypoxia and results in a marked shortening of action potential duration and rapid loss of contractile activity, Noma [1] proposed that these channels may play an important cardioprotective role. Indeed, since the subsequent development of selective modulators of this channel (that is, the K channel openers such as nicorandil, cromakalim, bimakalim, and aprikalim [4]) and the K_{ATP} channel antagonists (namely, the sulfonylurea antidiabetic agents, such as glibenclamide and tolbutamide [5], and the nonsulfonylurea agent, sodium 5-hydroxydecanoate [6]), considerable evidence has been obtained that suggests opening these channels is cardioprotective, while blocking these channels is proischemic and may actually delay the subsequent recovery of myocardial contractile function or result in an increase in the ultimate extent of myocardial infarction following ischemia and reperfusion [7–10]. The results of these studies support the original hypothesis of Noma [1], which suggested that opening of the K_{ATP} channel during ischemia is an endogenous cardioprotective mechanism, particularly in the early minutes of ischemia and during brief periods of ischemia followed by reperfusion. Since preconditioning is also produced by brief periods of ischemia and is an endogenous cardioprotective mechanism [11], it seemed reasonable to hypothesize that K_{ATP} channel opening may be an important component of this fascinating phenomenon. The following discussion will detail the evidence for and against a role for the K_{ATP} channel as a modulator in ischemic preconditioning in several animal models and species.

ROLE FOR K_{ATP} CHANNELS IN ISCHEMIC PRECONDITIONING IN DOGS

In the first report to describe a role for the K_{ATP} channel in ischemic preconditioning, our laboratory [12] found that intravenous administration of glibenclamide (a selective K_{ATP} channel antagonist), 10 minutes prior to or immediately upon reperfusion following the initial 5-minute ischemic period, completely abolished the beneficial effect of ischemic preconditioning in anesthetized dogs (Figure 1). The dose (0.3 mg/kg) of glibenclamide that was used produced a marked reduction in blood glucose levels but did not affect infarct size in nonpreconditioned control dogs. Intravenous infusion of a nonhypotensive dose of the selective K_{ATP} channel opener, aprikalim, produced a marked reduction in infarct size similar to that produced by preconditioning (see Figure 1). That glibenclamide blocked the effect of preconditioning when administered either prior to or after the preconditioning period suggests that K_{ATP} channel opening is involved in not only triggering preconditioning, but also in sustaining the protective effect into the prolonged ischemic episode.

Since intravenous administration of glibenclamide produced an increase in blood insulin levels and a marked decrease in blood glucose values, it is possible that an indirect metabolic effect of glibenclamide on the heart, independent of its action to block myocardial K_{ATP} channels, may have contributed to its effect on ischemic preconditioning. Accordingly, Auchampach et al. [13] infused the nonsulfonylurea K_{ATP} channel blocker so-

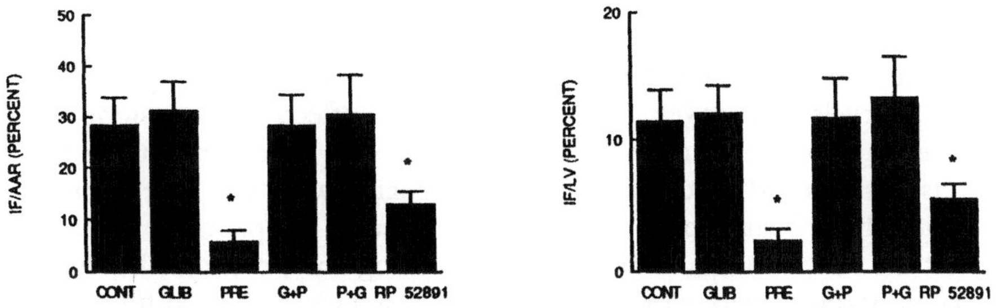

Figure 1. Graphs illustrating the effects of different treatments on infarct size (IF) expressed as a percent (IF/AAR) of the area at risk (AAR) or as a percent (IF/LV) of the left ventricle (LV) in the dog model. Preconditioning (PRE) and the selective potassium channel opener RP 52891 (RP, aprikalim) produced a significant reduction (*$p < 0.05$) in infarct size compared to the control nonpreconditioned group (CONT). Treatment with glibenclamide, a selective K_{ATP} antagonist, 10 minutes before (G+P) or immediately after (P+G) preconditioning, completely abolished its protective effect. Glibenclamide had no effect on infarct size in the absence of preconditioning (GLIB). Reprinted by permission from the American Heart Association, from Gross and Auchampach [12].

dium 5-hydroxydecanoate or small doses of glibenclamide directly into the coronary artery in nonpreconditioned and preconditioned dogs, thereby avoiding systemic metabolic effects due to changes in insulin and blood glucose. We found that preconditioning was completely blocked by both compounds (Figure 2), independent of changes in blood glucose and without

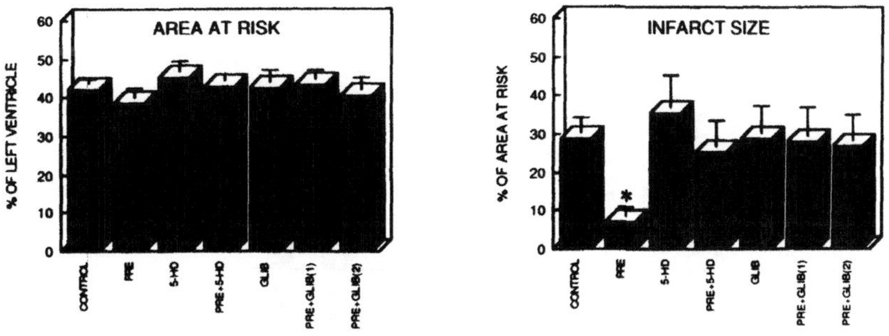

Figure 2. Graphs illustrating the effects of different treatments on the area at risk expressed as a percent of the left ventricle, and infarct size expressed as a percent of the area at risk in the dog model. There were no differences between groups in area at risk, however, preconditioning (PRE) produced a significant reduction in infarct size (*$p < 0.05$) as compared to he control nonpreconditioned group (CONTROL). Treatment with sodium 5-hydroxydecanoate (PRE+5HD) during both the preconditioning occlusion and the first 5 minutes of the 60-minute occlusion period abolished the protective effect of preconditioning. Similarly, in preconditioned dogs, treatment with glibenclamide (GLIB), either during the 5-minute preconditioning occlusion [PRE+GLIB(1)] or the first 5 minutes of the 60-minute occlusion [PRE+GLIB(2)], abolished the protective effect of preconditioning on infarct size. Neither 5-HD nor glibenclamide had an effect on infarct size in the absence of preconditioning. Reprinted by permission from the British Medical Journal Publishing Group, from Auchampach et al. [13].

any effect on infarct size in nonpreconditioned dogs. In agreement, Grover et al. [14] recently found that intracoronary glibenclamide also blocked preconditioning in anesthetized dogs, independent of changes in blood glucose levels. Moreover, the cardioprotective effects of potassium channel openers are unlikely to be related to changes in blood insulin or glucose levels, since most potassium channel openers, with the exception of diazoxide, have been shown to exert little effect on the pancreas at doses that affect the vasculature and heart [15]. Taken together, these results suggest a very important role for the K_{ATP} channel in ischemic preconditioning in the dog.

ROLE FOR K_{ATP} CHANNELS IN ISCHEMIC PRECONDITIONING IN PIGS

Recent preliminary results reported by Rohmann et al. [16] showed that intravenous administration of glibenclamide (1.0 mg/kg) blocked the beneficial effect of a 10-minute preconditioning episode in swine hearts (Figure

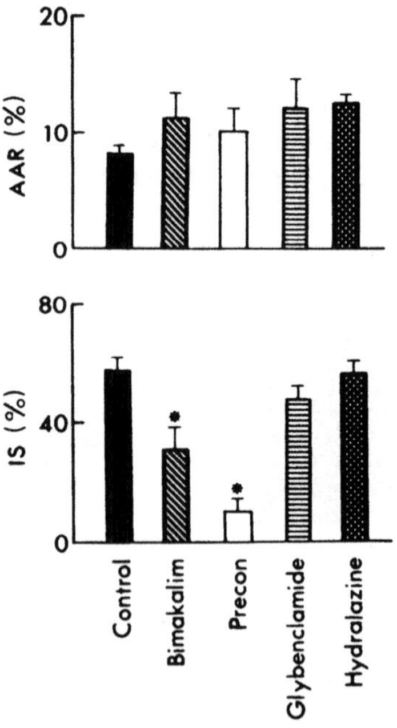

Figure 3. Graphs illustrating the effects of different treatments on the area at risk (AAR) expressed as a percent of the left ventricle and infarct size (IS) expressed as a percent of the area at risk in the swine model. Preconditioning (Precon) and the selective potassium channel opener bimakalim produced a significant reduction ($^*p < 0.05$) in infarct size as compared with the control nonpreconditioned group. Treatment with glibenclamide prior to preconditioning completely abolished its protective effect. Hydralazine, a vasodilator without K_{ATP} channel opening properties, had no effect on infarct size. Reprinted by permission from Rohmann et al. (personal communication, see Rohmann et al. [16]).

3). In addition, pretreatment of ischemic pig hearts with the selective K_{ATP} opener bimakalim produced a marked decrease in infarct size, although the reduction was not as great as that seen with preconditioning. Thus, these results suggest an important role for the K_{ATP} channel in ischemic preconditioning in pigs similar to that observed in dog hearts. Obviously, further studies are needed by other laboratories using this swine model to confirm these interesting preliminary results.

ROLE FOR THE K_{ATP} CHANNEL IN ISCHEMIC PRECONDITIONING IN RABBITS

The importance of the K_{ATP} channel in ischemic preconditioning in rabbits is equivocal. Recent results reported by Thornton et al. [17] suggest that activation of the K_{ATP} channel is not involved. These investigators showed that three doses (0.15, 0.30, and 3.0 mg/kg, iv) of glibenclamide produced significant increases in infarct size in the absence of preconditioning in rabbits, but did not block the beneficial effect of a 5-minute preconditioning episode. They also found that two doses of the K_{ATP} opener pinacidil did not reduce infarct size. In contrast, preliminary results of Toombs et al. (personal communication) showed that glibenclamide completely blocked the effect of ischemic preconditioning in rabbits at a dose (0.3 mg/kg) that did not increase infarct size in the absence of preconditioning (Figure 4). Toombs et al. [18] also showed that the K_{ATP} opener, cromakalim, reduced infarct size in rabbit hearts. Since both of these experiments in rabbits were performed using the same experimental protocol for preconditioning, the reason for the diametrically opposite results is not clear. The only apparent difference in the two studies relates to the anesthetic used. Thornton et al. [17] used pentobarbital anesthesia, whereas Toombs et al. [18] used xylazine and ketamine. Since pentobarbital has recently been shown to block the K_{ATP} channel [19], it is possible that the results obtained by Thornton et al. [17] may have been affected by use of this particular barbiturate. However, future experiments are needed to furnish a definitive answer as to the role of anesthesia and the K_{ATP} channel in ischemic preconditioning in rabbits.

ROLE FOR THE K_{ATP} CHANNEL IN ISCHEMIC PRECONDITIONING IN RATS

Several recent reports [20,21] suggest that the K_{ATP} channel is not involved in ischemic preconditioning in rat hearts. Liu and Downey [20] showed that three 5-minute cycles of preconditioning protected the rat heart from a subsequent infarction, and that pretreatment with the K_{ATP} channel antagonist glibenclamide did not block the protective effect of preconditioning (Figure 5). Grover et al. [21] also showed that glibenclamide, even at concentrations of up to 100 μM, did not attenuate the ability of ischemic preconditioning to enhance the recovery of left ventricular developed pressure in isolated buffer-perfused rat hearts. Although the end point in this latter study

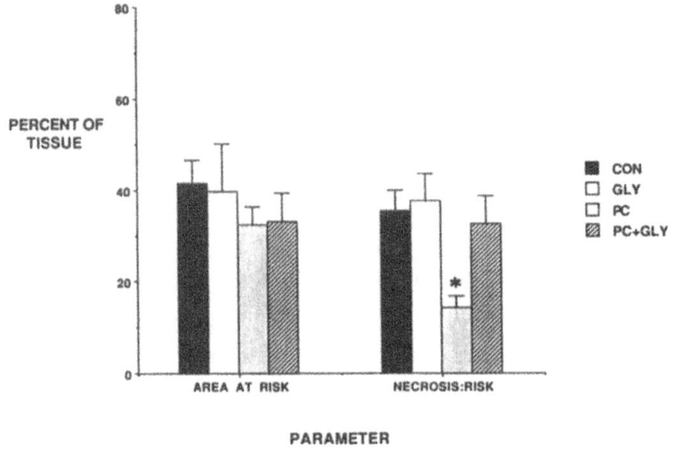

Figure 4. Graph illustrating the effect of different treatments on the area at risk as a percent of the left ventricle and infarct size (NECROSIS) as a percent of the area at risk in the rabbit model. There were no differences among groups in area at risk, however, preconditioning (PC) produced a significant (*$p < 0.05$) reduction in infarct size as compared to the control nonpreconditioned group (CON). Pretreatment with glibenclamide (GLY) completely abolished the protective effect of preconditioning (PC+GLY). Glibenclamide (GLY) had no effect on infarct size in the absence of preconditioning. Reprinted by permission from Toombs et al. (personal communication).

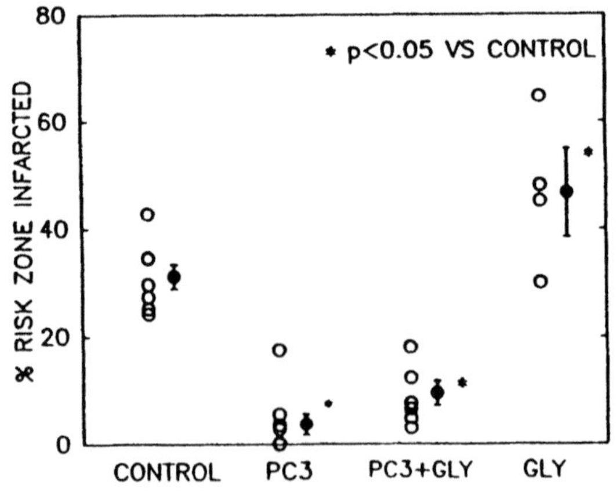

Figure 5. Infarct size in rat hearts preconditioned in situ are shown for control, preconditioned (PC3) and glibenclamide-treated (GLY) groups. Filled symbol in each group indicates group mean ± SE; open symbols indicate infarct sizes from individual hearts (*$p < 0.05$ vs. control). Reprinted by permission from the American Physiological Society from Liu and Downey [20]).

[21] was not infarction, these results are similar to those of Liu and Downey [20] in that neither study supports a role for the K_{ATP} channel in ischemic preconditioning in this species. On the other hand, Grover et al. [22,23] have clearly demonstrated that several K channel openers are cardioprotective in the isolated rat heart, and Liu and Downey [20] showed an increase in infarct size in the presence of glibenclamide. Thus, it appears that the K_{ATP} channel does serve an important cardioprotective role in this species in spite of the negative findings in preconditioned hearts.

INTERACTION BETWEEN ADENOSINE AND THE K_{ATP} CHANNEL IN ISCHEMIC PRECONDITIONING

Initially, Kirsch et al. [24] showed that activation of adenosine A_1 receptors in neonatal rat ventricular myocytes opens the K_{ATP} channel via stimulation of a G_i protein. Similarly, lto et al. [25] found that adenosine activated the K_{ATP} channel in guinea pig ventricular myocytes via the $G_{i\alpha}$ subunit of the G_i protein. Since there is evidence (albeit equivocal) that suggests adenosine acting via its A_1 receptor triggers ischemic preconditioning [26,27] in several species, it seems reasonable to hypothesize that part of its beneficial effect may be mediated via K_{ATP} channel activation. In support of this hypothesis, Grover et al. [14] recently found that a selective A_1 receptor agonist R-phenyl isopropyl adenosine(R-PIA) produced a reduction in infarct size similar to that produced by ischemic preconditioning in dogs, and that this beneficial effect was abolished by glibenclamide. Similarly, Auchampach et al. [26] showed that a 5-minute intracoronary infusion of adenosine plus a small dose of dipyridamole reduced infarct size in dogs, and found that this effect was also blocked by glibenclamide. Preliminary results obtained in pigs by Van Winkle et al. [28] showed that the antiinfarct effect of R-PIA was blocked by sodium 5-hydroxydeconoate, another selective blocker of the K_{ATP} channel. Taken together, these data all support the original findings of Kirsch et al. [24] and Ito et al. [25], and further suggest that the ability of adenosine and/or ischemic preconditioning to protect the heart during a more prolonged ischemic insult may be mediated via an A_1 receptor-G_i mediated opening of the K_{ATP} channel. In support of a role for a G_i protein, Thornton and Downey [29] recently showed that pertussis toxin blocked the effect of preconditioning in rabbit hearts. Obviously, more studies are needed in the rabbit and rat to confirm or reject the hypothesis that the protective effect of adenosine A_1 receptor stimulation and ischemic preconditioning is mediated via K_{ATP} channel activation.

MECHANISM(S) RESPONSIBLE FOR THE PROTECTIVE EFFECT OF ISCHEMIC PRECONDITIONING VIA K_{ATP} CHANNEL OPENING

The mechanism by which K_{ATP} channel activation mediates the effect of ischemic preconditioning is currently not clear. Noma [1] originally hypothesized that activation of the K_{ATP} channel would lead to a shortening of action potential duration, a decrease in calcium influx, a rapid loss of contractile function, and an energy-sparing effect, which would reduce the rate of ATP depletion. Several studies in the isolated rat heart [22,23], guinea pig right ventricular free wall [7], and in situ canine heart [10,30] support this hypothesis. D'Alonso et al. [10], Mitani et al. [31], Galinanes et al. [32], and Yao and Gross [30] have shown that K_{ATP} channel openers accelerate the ischemia-induced shortening of action potential duration, increase the rate of loss of contractile activity, and preserve ATP levels in several animal models of ischemia-reperfusion injury.

If the K_{ATP} channel is involved in ischemic preconditioning, the activity of this channel would need to be increased or primed by the initial preconditioning insult so that it would open more rapidly or to a greater extent during the subsequent more prolonged ischemic insult. Although this hypothesis has not been clearly tested experimentally, adenosine, acting via its A_1 receptor, might be a possible candidate for this priming agent, since this compound has been shown to activate the K_{ATP} channel via a G_i-mediated mechanism in several species [24,25]. Whether adenosine decreases the sensitivity of the channel to ATP during the second prolonged ischemic insult and increases K_{ATP} activity is currently unknown, but might be a potential mechanism to explain the phenomenon of ischemic preconditioning [33].

Another potential candidate for maintaining K_{ATP} channel activity following a brief ischemic insult is protein kinase C. DeWeille et al. [34] have

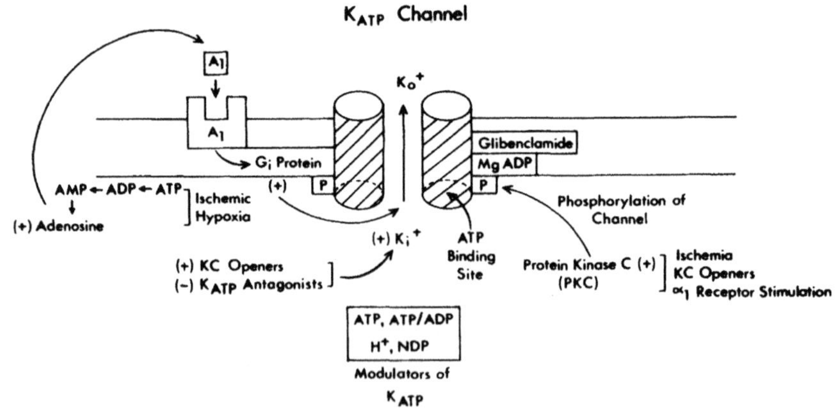

Figure 6. A schematic drawing of the ATP-sensitive potassium channel (K_{ATP}) and the possible interrelationships between the adenosine A_1 receptor and the G_i protein, protein kinase C (PKC), and the K_{ATP} channel. Other factors that modulate the K_{ATP} channel are shown, such as ATP, the ATP/ADP ratio, H^+, nucleotide diphosphates (NDP), potassium channel (KC) openers, and K_{ATP} antagonists. The three proposed binding sites for ATP, MgADP, and glibenclamide are also represented. The hypothesized site for PKC-mediated membrane phosphorylation (P) is also shown. (+) represents a stimulatory response and (−) represents an inhibitory response.

recently shown that in rat insulinoma cells, stimulation of protein kinase C by somatostatin or the phorbol ester, phorbol myristate acetate (PMA), activates the K_{ATP} channel. It has also been recently demonstrated that a brief 5-minute period of ischemia is sufficient to activate protein kinase C [35], and Downey reported at the 1992 American Heart Association meetings that activation of protein kinase C may be involved in ischemic preconditioning in rabbit hearts (personal communication). Thus, although speculative, it is possible that protein kinase C activation might prolong or enhance K_{ATP} channel opening by phosphorylating a membrane protein involved in maintaining K_{ATP} channel opening (Figure 6).

SUMMARY AND CLINICAL IMPLICATIONS

Considerable evidence currently exists that suggests an important role for activation of the K_{ATP} channel in ischemic preconditioning in dogs and pigs; the evidence supporting a role for this channel is equivocal in rabbits and negative in rat hearts. However, in all species tested, the majority of evidence suggests that opening of the K_{ATP} channel is antiischemic, whereas blocking the channel is proischemic. Whether this channel is an important mediator of ischemic preconditioning in all animal species, and the mechanism by which the K_{ATP} channel produces a cardioprotective effect, both await further experimentation. If this is found to be the case, potassium channel openers such as aprikalim, bimakalim, or cromakalim may be useful drugs in clinical applications where stimulating or mimicking ischemic preconditioning may be a desirable goal.

These results may also have important clinical implications, since a significant number of patients with non-insulin-dependent diabetes are currently taking sulfonylurea antidiabetic drugs, which are potent blockers of the K_{ATP} channel. Blockade of these channels in the myocardium may render these patients susceptible to an increased risk of injury during single or multiple ischemic episodes, as are known to occur in unstable angina or myocardial infarction. In support of this possibility, the results of a previous study published more than 20 years ago [36] suggested that patients with adult onset diabetes had a higher mortality rate from cardiovascular disease when receiving tolbutamide than those receiving placebo or insulin. Whether these results can be explained by an effect of tolbutamide to block preconditioning in human hearts is unknown, but represents an interesting possibility.

ACKNOWLEDGMENTS

The authors wish to thank Jeanine Moore, Anna Hsu, and Aileen Fiorita for excellent technical assistance, artwork, and typing in the preparation of this manuscript. The research results reported from the authors' laboratory were supported by USPHS grant HL 08311.

REFERENCES

1. Noma A. 1983. ATP-regulated K^+ channels in cardiac muscle. Nature 305:147–148.
2. Gross GJ, Auchampach JA. 1992. Role of ATP dependent potassium channels in myocardial ischemia. Cardiovasc Res 26:1011–1016.
3. Nichols CG, Lederer WJ. 1991. Adenosine triphosphate-sensitive potassium channels in the cardiovascular system. Am J Physiol 262:H1675–1686.
4. Edwards G, Weston AH. 1990. Structure-activity relationships of K^+ channel openers. Trends Pharmacol Sci 11:417–422.
5. Sturgess NC, Ashford ML, Cook DL, Hales CN. 1985. The sulfonylurea receptor may be an ATP-sensitive potassium channel. Lancet 2:474–475.
6. McCullough JR, Normandin DE, Condor ML, Sleph PG, Dzwonczyk S, Grover GJ. 1991. Specific block of the anti-ischemic actions of cromakalim by sodium 5-hydroxydecanoate. Circ Res 69:949–958.
7. Cole WG, McPherson CD, Sontag D. 1991. ATP-regulated K^+ channels protect the myocardium against ischemia/reperfusion damage. Circ Res 69:571–581.
8. Auchampach JA, Maruyama M, Cavero I, Gross GJ. 1991. The new K^+ channel opener RP 52891 reduces experimental infarct size in dogs in the absence of systemic hemodynamic changes. J Pharmacol Exp Ther 259:961–967.
9. Auchampach JA, Maruyama M, Cavero I, Gross GJ. 1992. Pharmacological evidence for a role of ATP-regulated potassium channels in myocardial stunning. Circulation 86:311–319.
10. D'Alonso AJ, Darbenzio RB, Parham CS, Grover GJ. 1992. Effects of intracoronary cromakalim on postischemic contractile function and action potential duration. Cardiovase Res 26:1046–1053.
11. Murry CE, Jennings RB, Reimer KA. 1986. Preconditioning with ischemia: A delay of lethal cell injury in ischemic myocardium. Circulation 74:1124–1136.
12. Gross, GJ, Auchampach JA. 1992. Blockade of ATP-sensitive potassium channels prevents myocardial preconditioning in dogs. Circ Res 70:223–233.
13. Auchampach JA, Grover GJ, Gross GJ. 1992. Blockade of ischemic preconditioning in dogs by the novel ATP dependent potassium channel antagonist sodium 5–hydroxydecanoate. Cardiovasc Res 26:1054–1062.
14. Grover, GJ, Sleph PG, Dzwonczyk S. 1992. Role of myocardial ATP-sensitive potassium channels in mediating preconditioning in the dog heart and their possible interaction with adenosine A_1 receptors. Circulation 86:1310–1316.
15. Lebrun P, Antoine MH, Herchuelz A. 1992. Minireview: K^+ channel openers and insulin release. Life Sci 51:795–806.
16. Rohmann SM, Weygandt H, Schelling P, Lues I. 1992. ATP-sensitive potassium channel (K_{ATP}) opener bimakalim mimics preconditioning in swine. Circulation 86(Suppl 4):I555.
17. Thornton JD, Thornton CS, Sterling DL, Downey JM. 1993. Blockade of ATP-sensitive potassium channels increases infarct size but does not prevent preconditioning in rabbit hearts. Circ Res 72:44–49.
18. Toombs CF, Norman NR, Groppi VE, Lee KS, Gadwood RC, Shebuski RJ. 1992. Limitation of myocardial injury with the potassium channel opener cromakalim and the nonvasoactive analog U-89,232: vascular vs. cardiac actions in vitro and in vivo. J Pharmacol Exp Ther 263:1261–1268.
19. Kozlowski RZ, Ashford MLJ. 1991. Barbiturates inhibit ATP-K^+ channels and voltage-activated currents in CRI-GI insulin-secreting cells. Br J Pharmacol 103:2021–2029.
20. Liu Y, Downey JM. 1992. Ischemic preconditioning protects against infarction in rat heart. Am J Physiol 263:H1107–H1112.
21. Grover GJ, Dzwonczyk S, Sleph PG. 1992. ATP-sensitive K^+ channel activation does not mediate preconditioning in isolated rat hearts. Circulation 86(Suppl 4):I341.
22. Grover GJ, McCullough JR, Henry DE, Condor ML, Sleph PG. 1989. The anti-ischemic effects of the potassium channel activators pinacidil and cromakalim and the reversal of these effects with the potassium channel blocker glyburide. J Pharmacol Exp Ther 251: 98–110.
23. Grover GJ, Dwonczyk S, Parham CS, Sleph PG. 1990. The protective effect of cromakalim and pinacidil on reperfusion function and infarct size in isolated rat hearts and anesthetized dogs. Cardiovas Drugs Ther 15:465–474.

24. Kirsch GE, Codina J, Birnbaumer L, Brown AM. 1990. Coupling of ATP-sensitive K^+ channels to A_1 receptors by G proteins in rat ventricular myocytes. Am J Physiol 259:H820–H826.
25. Ito H, Tung RT, Sugimoto T, Kobayashi I, Takahashi K, Katada T, Ui M, Kurachi Y. 1992. On the mechanism of G protein by subunit activation of the muscarinic K^+ channel in guinea pig atrial cell membrane: Comparison with the ATP-sensitive K^+ channel. J Gen Physiol 99:961–983.
26. Auchampach JA, Gross GJ. 1992. Activation of ATP-dependent (K_{ATP}) channels by adenosine: A possible mechanism for ischemic preconditioning in dogs. Circulation 86(Suppl 4):I340.
27. Liu GS, Thornton J, Van Winkle DM, Stanley AWH, Olsson RA, Downey JM. 1991. Protection against infarction afforded by preconditioning is mediated via A_1 adenosine receptors in rabbit heart. Circulation 84:350–356.
28. Van Winkle DM, Chien GL, Wolff RA, Soifer BE, Davis RF. 1992. Intracoronary infusion of R-phenyl isopropyl adenosine prior to ischemia/reperfusion reduces myocardial infarct size in swine. Circulation 86(Suppl 4):I213.
29. Thornton J, Downey JM. 1991. G_i proteins are involved in preconditioning's protective effects. Circulation 84(Suppl 4):II192.
30. Yao Z, Cavero I, Gross GJ. 1993. Activation of cardiac K_{ATP} channels: An endogenous protective mechanism during repetitive ischemia. Am J Physiol, in press.
31. Mitani A, Kinoshita K, Fukamachi K, Sakamoto M, Kurisu K, Tsuruhara Y, Fukumura F, Nakashima A, Tokunaga K. 1991. Effects of glibenclamide and nicorandil on cardiac function during ischemia and reperfusion in isolated perfused rat hearts. Am J Physiol 261:H1864–H1871.
32. Galinanes M, Shattock MJ, Hearse DJ. 1992. Effects of potassium channel modulation during global ischaemia in isolated rat heart with and without cardioplegia. Cardiovasc Res 26:1063–1068.
33. Walker, DM, Yellon DM. 1992. Ischaemic preconditioning: From mechanisms to exploitation. Cardiovasc Res 26:734–739.
34. DeWeille JR, Schmid-Antomarchi H, Fosset M, Lazdunski M. 1989. Regulation of ATP-sensitive K^+ channels in insulinoma cells: Activation by somatostatin and protein kinase C and the role of cAMP. Proc Natl Acad Sci USA 86:2971–2975.
35. Strasser RH, Braun-Dullaeus R, Walendzik H, Marquetant R 1992. α_1-Receptor-independent activation of protein kinase C in acute myocardial infarction. Circ Res 70:1304–1312.
36. Meinart Cl, Knatlerud GL, Prout TE. 1970. A study of the effects of hypoglycemic agents on vascular complications in patients with adult-onset diabetes. Diabetes 19:747–830.

8. ADENOSINE AND THE ANTIINFARCT EFFECTS OF PRECONDITIONING

JAMES M. DOWNEY, YONGGE LIU, and KIRSTI YTREHUS

INTRODUCTION

Preconditioning the myocardium with a brief period of ischemia followed by reperfusion causes it to become very resistant to both infarction [1–4] and, in some models, arrhythmias [5–7] from a subsequent more prolonged ischemia. Ischemic preconditioning is the most potent protector against ischemia known for the heart and has received widespread confirmation as to its efficacy. The mechanism of this protection has been elusive, but there is mounting evidence from this and other laboratories that adenosine plays an important role in the antiinfarct effect, at least in some species. During even the briefest coronary occlusion, adenosine is produced and released by the heart [8]. While adenosine has been the focus of cardiovascular studies for many years, adenosine has only recently been proposed to be directly cardioprotective independent of its vascular effects. This concept was first proposed by Ely and colleagues [9], and today the number of papers describing adenosine-mediated protection appears to be increasing geometrically. This chapter will review the evidence that the cellular changes associated with the preconditioning phenomenon are triggered by adenosine released during the preconditioning ischemia.

ADENOSINE HYPOTHESIS

We [10] and others [11] have shown that as little as 5 minutes of coronary occlusion can fully invoke the antiinfarct effect of preconditioning and that this protection persisted for 15–30 minutes [3,10]. Adenosine is released in large quantity within seconds after the onset of myocardial ischemia [8] as catabolism of ATP exceeds production. During ischemia, adenosine levels reach the micromolar range [12], which is more than sufficient to populate cardiac receptors.

In light of adenosine's reported protective effects [9], it seemed plausible that adenosine receptor occupancy during the preconditioning ischemia could have triggered the protective changes. We therefore tested the adenosine hypothesis in a series of experiments using the anesthetized, open-chest rabbit model of myocardial infarction. In this model, a branch of the left coronary artery is ligated for 30 minutes and then reperfused for several hours. Infarct size is determined by staining the hearts with triphenyl tetrazolium chloride (TTC), an accurate method of assessing ultimate infarct size in this model [13]. As rabbits lack preformed coronary collateral vessels, we believe that it is not necessary to incorporate collateral flow as a covariant in the infarct size analysis, as is the case in dog studies [14,15].

Adenosine receptor blockers block the antiinfarct effect of preconditioning

In a recent report [16] we tested two broad-acting adenosine receptor blockers, 8-p-sulfophenyl theophylline (SPT) and N-[2-(dimethylamino) ethyl] Nmethyl-4-(2,3,6,7-tetrahydro-2,6-dioxo-1,3-dipropyl-1H-purin-8-yl) benzosulfonamide (PD 115,199). The blockers were given 5 minutes prior to a 5-minute preconditioning ischemia. The hearts were then reperfused for 10 minutes prior to a 30-minute ischemic insult. The study design consisted of both ischemically preconditioned and nonpreconditioned (control) rabbits .

Figure 1 (left panel) reveals that 38% of the ischemic tissue (risk zone) was infarcted in the unblocked and nonpreconditioned control group. Preconditioning the control hearts caused significant protection from infarction, with infarct size averaging only 9% of the risk zone. Pretreatment with SPT (middle panel) resulted in 53% infarction in nonpreconditioned hearts, which, although larger, did not achieve significance against the unblocked control infarct size. *SPT blocked the protective effect of preconditioning: 39% of the ischemic zone became infarcted, which did not differ significantly from that seen in the nonpreconditioned hearts.*

Pretreatment with another blocker having a different chemical structure, PD 115,199, also blocked the protective effect of preconditioning (Figure 1, right panel). Virgin hearts pretreated with PD 115,199 developed 46% infarction, and preconditioned hearts pretreated with PD 115,199 exhibited 38% infarction. Again the infarct sizes in both groups blocked with PD 115,199 were not different from that in the unblocked control group.

Preconditioning can be triggered by exogenous adenosine

The ability of the adenosine receptor blockers to block preconditioning confirmed our suspicion that the occupation of adenosine receptors is in-

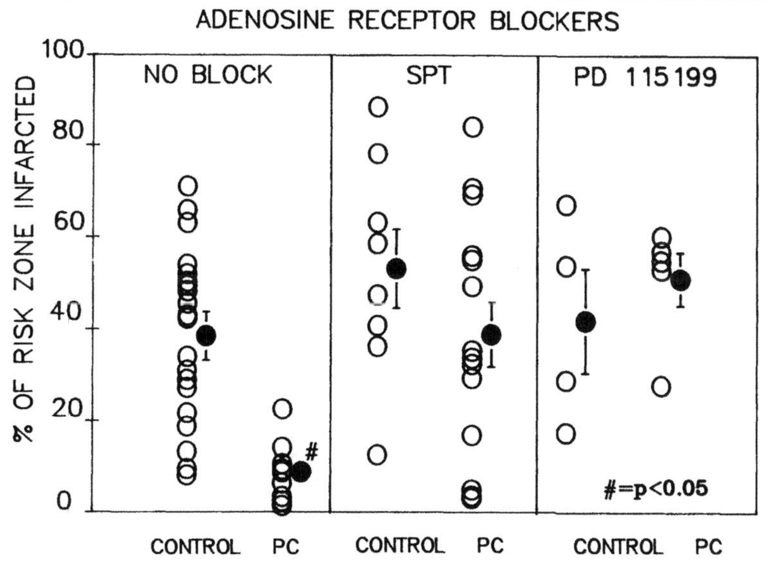

Figure 1. Infarct size, expressed as a percentage of the risk zone, appears on the vertical axis. Open symbols represent individual animals, and closed symbols are means and standard error for the groups. Preconditioning (PC) the heart with 5 minutes of ischemia protects it against infarction. But either of the adenosine receptor blockers 8-p-sulfophenyl theophylline (SPT) or N-[2-(dimethylamino) ethyl] N-methyl-4-(2,3,6,7-tetrahydro-2,6-dioxo-1,3-dipropyl-1H-purin-8-yl) benzosulfonamide (PD 115 199) block that protection but have little effect on the nonpreconditioned heart. Reproduced with permission from Liu et al. [16].

volved in the protective effect. If the hypothesis that endogenous adenosine released during the brief ischemia was the initiator of preconditioning, then exposure of the heart to exogenous adenosine should protect the heart as well as exposure to ischemia.

To test this hypothesis we wanted to infuse adenosine directly into the coronary arteries to avoid profound systemic vasodilation. Since intracoronary injections are technically impossible for us to perform in the rabbit, a blood-perfused isolated heart model was used [16]. The hearts were all electrically paced to avoid the bradycardia associated with intracoronary adenosine. The hearts underwent 45 minutes of regional ischemia followed by 2 hours of reperfusion to induce an infarct. Figure 2 (second column) reveals that these isolated hearts could still be protected by an ischemic preconditioning protocol (5 minutes ischemia + 10 minutes reperfusion). In a third group, adenosine was added directly into the coronary perfusate for 5 minutes at a total dose of 1.4 mg. The infusion was then stopped for 10 minutes to simulate the period of reperfusion. As shown in Figure 2 (third column) *intracoronary adenosine protected the isolated heart to the same degree as preconditioning*.

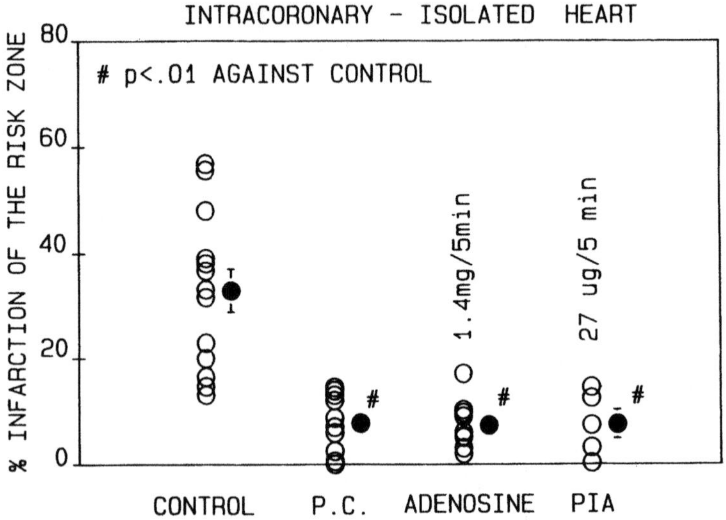

Figure. 2. Intracoronary infusion of adenosine or the A_1-selective agonist, N^6-(phenyl-2R-isopropyl)-adenosine (PIA), was equipotent with ischemic preconditioning (P.C.) in protecting the isolated blood perfused rabbit heart from infarction. Reproduced with permission from Liu et al. [16].

PROTECTION IS VIA THE A_1 ADENOSINE RECEPTOR

We determined which adenosine receptor subtype was initiating the preconditioning protection by using the A_1 selective analog N^6-(phenyl-2R-isopropyl)-adenosine, rPIA. The fourth column of Figure 2 reveals that rPIA also protected the isolated heart when infused at a total dose of 27 μg over 5 minutes [16]. The dose of rPIA was chosen because it lengthened the P–R interval, an A_1 adenosine receptor effect, but had no effect on the coronary resistance, an A_2 adenosine receptor effect. Recently Van Winkle et al. [17] gave rPIA (2.5 μg/kg/min) into the coronary arteries of pigs prior to an ischemic insult and again saw a dramatic reduction of infarct size. A similar antiinfarct effect was seen when rPIA (0.4 μg/kg/min) was infused into the coronary artery of dogs [18]. *Because the A_1-selective agonist appeared to be equipotent with preconditioning, we concluded that the A_1 adenosine receptor is responsible for the reduction in infarct size associated with preconditioning.*

A_1-selective adenosine analogs are protective when administered intravenously

We have been unable to trigger the protection with parenteral administration of adenosine [16]. A dose of 5 mg/min for 5 minutes of adenosine produced profound hypotension and further increases in dose were not tolerated by the animals. Infarct size in this group was 44% of the area at risk, which was not different from that in the control group. *The inability of intravenous adenosine to protect could have been due to our failure to provide a sufficient concentration of adenosine to the myocardium.* In particular, adenosine deaminase activity in the blood and lungs quickly degrades adenosine, which would limit the amount of adenosine that actually gets to the heart. This theory was supported by the fact that no slowing of the heart rate, a known cardiac effect of adenosine, was seen with intravenous (iv) adenosine. Others, however, have observed preconditioning with iv adenosine. Toombs et al. reported that an iv infusion of only 140 μg/kg/min of adenosine prior to ischemia caused a 70% reduction of infarct size in the rabbit model [19]. We have no explanation for the discrepant data, other than perhaps the outcome was influenced by the different anesthetic agents; i.e., we used pentobarbital while Toombs et al. used ketamine-xylazine.

In our hands, hypotension (assumed to be an A_2 effect) limited our ability to administer an adequate dose of intravenous adenosine. We, therefore, tested whether an A_1-selective agonist might be protective when given intravenously, since it should not cause peripheral dilation. Three adenosine analogs were tested: rPIA, which is about 100-fold selective for A_1 receptor; 2-chloro-N^6-cyclopentyladenosine (CCPA), which is 10,000-fold A_1 selective, and 2-[4-(2-carboxyethyl)phenethylamino]-5′-N-ethylcarboxamido adenosine hydrochloride (CGS 21680), a 170-fold A_2-selective agonist. All of the animals were subjected to a 30-minute coronary occlusion followed by 180 minutes of reperfusion.

We gave a 5-minute iv infusion of rPIA (915 μg/kg) beginning 15 minutes before a 30-minute occlusion. The second column in Figure 3 reveals that only 7% of the ischemic region infarcted with iv rPIA (the "PIA-no pace" group). When the same dose of rPIA was given just prior to reperfusion after a single 30-minute occlusion (column 3 in Figure 3), no protection was realized (45% infarction), indicating that A_1 receptor occupancy must precede ischemia in order to limit infarct size.

A_1 agonists cause a profound reduction in heart rate. To test whether the bradycardia caused by rPIA was responsible for the protection, we eliminated the decrease in heart rate with pacing. We infused 915 μg/kg rPIA before ischemia and paced at 200 beats/min beginning at the onset of drug infusion. Only 16% of the risk region infarcted (rPIA paced group in Figure 3), indicating that the bradycardia was not responsible for the protection.

We next tested the highly A_1-selective agonist, CCPA [20]. Rabbits received 250 μg/kg iv of CCPA 15 minutes prior to the 30-minute ischemic period. Figure 3 (column 5) reveals that CCPA was also very protective, with only 10% of the ischemic zone becoming necrotic. We have recently confirmed that iv CCPA induces a sustained limitation of infarct size in a 3-day reperfusion model [21]. Tsuchida et al. saw a similar result when iv rPIA was tested in the rabbit with an extended reperfusion period, although they had to counter the hypotension with pacing to achieve protec-

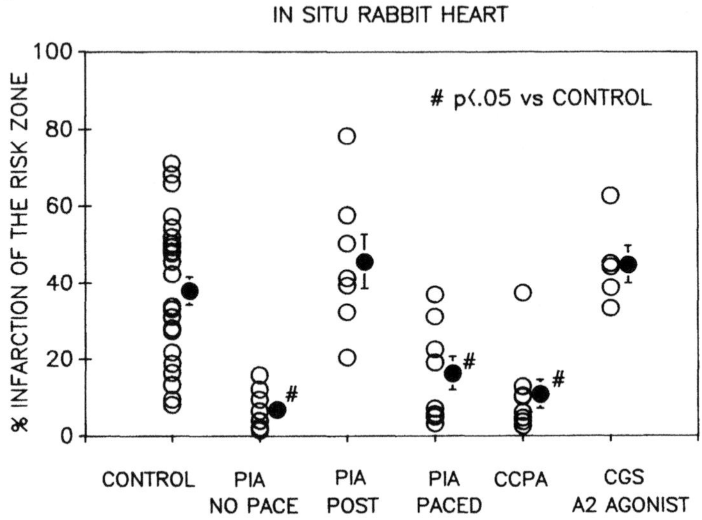

Figure 3. The effect of intravenous administration of receptor-selective adenosine analogs on infarct size following a 30-minute ischemic insult. PIA NO PACE refers to pretreatment with 915 μg/kg rPIA 15 minutes prior to coronary occlusion. PIA POST refers to injection of rPIA 2 minutes prior to reperfusion. PIA PACED refers to rPIA pretreatment with pacing at 220 beats/min to eliminate the bradycardia. CCPA refers to animals pretreated with 250 μg/kg 2-chloro-N^6-cyclopentyladenosine, a highly A_1-selective analog. CGS A2 AGONIST refers to animals pretreated with 80 μg/kg of CGS 21680, a highly A_2-selective adenosine analog. Reproduced with permission from Thornton et al. [23].

tion in that study [22]. When we gave the A_2-selective agonist, CGS 21680 at 80 μg/kg, 15 minutes prior to the 30-minute occlusion, no protection was seen (42% infarction, the last panel in Figure 3).

The hemodynamic results of the experiment are seen in Figure 4. As expected rPIA and CCPA reduced heart rate by about 30%, an A_1 effect [8]. All three analogs caused a marked decrease in mean arterial blood pressure [23]. Pacing the heart at the onset of rPIA infusion eliminated the decrease in heart rate but did not fully eliminate the hypotension. We also found that cardiac output was reduced with rPIA and CCPA, indicating that hypotension was a result of cardiac depression. Note that the A_2 agonist CGS 21680 had no effect on heart rate but caused a fall in arterial pressure to a level comparable to that seen with rPIA. The cardiac output in these animals was increased, revealing that the hypotension was due to A_2-mediated peripheral dilation rather than cardiac depression. All three agents caused prolonged hypotension, which lasted for the remainder of the study as none are rapidly metabolized. *We conclude that the intravenous administration of A_1-selective agonists does induce a real and sustained limitation of infarct size.*

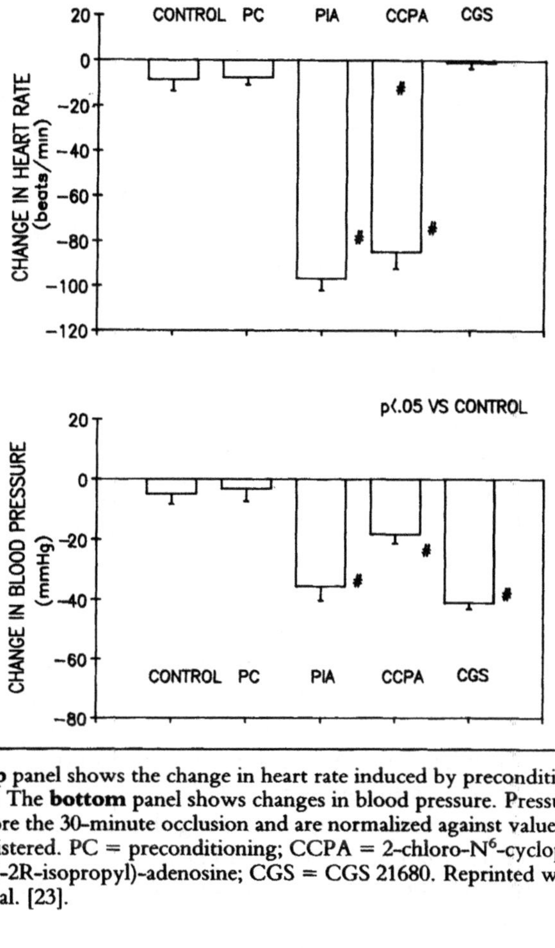

Figure 4. The **top** panel shows the change in heart rate induced by preconditioning or the three adenosine analogs. The **bottom** panel shows changes in blood pressure. Pressure and rates were measured just before the 30-minute occlusion and are normalized against values taken before drugs were administered. PC = preconditioning; CCPA = 2-chloro-N^6-cyclopentyladenosine; PIA = N^6-(phenyl-2R-isopropyl)-adenosine; CGS = CGS 21680. Reprinted with permission from Thornton et al. [23].

Adenosine promoter, acadesine, lowers the threshold for preconditioning

Further evidence that adenosine is the mediator of preconditioning can be derived from studies using adenosine promoters. These agents augment the adenosine levels in tissue, particularly when tissue becomes ischemic. To date acadesine (AICA riboside), dipyridamole, and R75231 have been studied in the infarct model [24–26]. No compound had an effect on infarct size in nonpreconditioned hearts but all lowered the threshold for preconditioning. Two minutes of ischemia, which is normally insufficient to induce the preconditioning phenomenon in rabbit heart, caused protection in hearts treated with these drugs. We believe that the threshold for protection was lowered as a result of increased adenosine release during the preconditioning ischemia.

Adenosine appears to both initiate and mediate preconditioning

The results from these studies support the hypothesis that preconditioning is triggered by A_1 adenosine receptor occupancy. When adenosine was infused into the coronary perfusate of the isolated heart, a 10-minute recovery period followed the adenosine infusion [16]. Adenosine has a very short half-life in tissues such that little of the infusate would have been present after 10 minutes, yet the protection persisted. Those results reinforced our belief that endogenous adenosine released during the preconditioning ischemia *triggers* an intracellular change that protects the heart during the subsequent ischemia.

Adenosine is released, however, not only during the preconditioning ischemia but also during the long ischemia. The question then arises: *Is occupancy of adenosine receptors important during the sustained ischemia?* The data would at first suggest that adenosine released during a prolonged ischemia is not important; i.e., when adenosine receptors are blocked prior to ischemia in virgin hearts, no significant exacerbation of infarction was seen (Figure 1). However, we chose to directly address this question by varying the time at which adenosine receptor blockade was initiated.

When we administered the adenosine receptor blocking agent, PD 115,199, after preconditioning with a 5-minute occlusion but prior to the 30-minute ischemic insult, protection was still blocked [27]. Toombs et al. saw a similar result when adenosine receptors were blocked following preconditioning with adenosine [19]. When the blocker PD 115,199 was administered at the end of the 30-minute sustained ischemia in preconditioned animals, the protective effect of preconditioning persisted (17% infarction, $p < 0.05$ vs. control, $p =$ ns vs. preconditioned), indicating that adenosine exerts its effect during ischemia rather than at reperfusion [27].

The fact that receptor occupancy is required during the long ischemia for protection to occur would suggest that adenosine is not only a *trigger* for preconditioning, but acts as a *mediator* of preconditioning as well. *These experiments reveal that the preconditioned heart behaves as if it had become sensitive to its own adenosine during the prolonged ischemia.*

The most likely explanation for the apparent mediator role of adenosine in the preconditioned heart is that an intracellular signalling pathway between the adenosine receptor and the end effector of the protection is acutely upregulated when the heart is in the preconditioned state. Furthermore, it appears that populating A_1 adenosine receptors is the trigger for that upregulation. Such behavior is counter to what is usually seen with receptor systems, where receptor stimulation usually leads to a desensitization of the signalling pathway rather than an upregulation. While the end effector in this pathway is currently unknown, recent studies have shed some light on the intracellular signalling pathways involved and are discussed below.

Another way that adenosine could mediate preconditioning is for the preconditioned heart to produce more adenosine during ischemia. Kitakaze et al. [28], using a dog model, reported that the preconditioned heart exhibited more 5′-nucleotidase activity and produced more adenosine that control animals. This increase in adenosine production via 5′-nucleotidase during the prolonged ischemia would also cause more adenosine receptor occupancy in preconditioned tissue and thus protect the heart. Kitakaze and colleagues also have evidence that ischemia, perhaps through adenosine release, triggers this increase in 5′ nucleotidase activity through intracellular signalling pathways involving a protein kinase C mechanism [29]. At present we do not know which, if any, of these theories are correct.

Long-term desensitization of A_1 receptors

We also examined the effect of long-term infusion of the A_1-selective analog, CCPA [30]. We infused CCPA at 0.43 μg/hr/kg for up to 72 hours. Six hours after the beginning of the infusion one group of the animals underwent a 30-minute regional ischemia followed by 2 hours of reperfusion. Bradycardia was present in treated rabbits (179 vs. 256 beats/min in control rabbits treated with vehicle) and infarcts were smaller in the treated group (16% infarction vs. 39% in the vehicle group), indicating that the hearts were still protected after a 6-hour infusion. That was not the case in the 72-hour infusion group, however. Following 72 hours of infusion, the heart rate had recovered to normal (247 vs. 264 beats/min in the vehicle group), indicating desensitization of the A_1 receptors had occurred. As expected, infarcts in the 72-hour CCPA infusion group after a 30-minute insult were no different from that in the 72-hour vehicle infusion group (37% infarction vs. 35% in vehicle). Similarly, a 5-minute ischemic preconditioning protocol in the desensitized group conferred little protection to these animals (29% infarction). These results, while confirming again the primacy of the A_1 receptor in preconditioning, indicate that *receptor desensitization would probably prevent long-term cardioprotection using an adenosine-based drug.*

ADENOSINE, PRECONDITIONING, AND G PROTEINS

A_1 adenosine receptors invariably have been found to be coupled to pertussis toxin-sensitive G-proteins [31,32]. If A_1 adenosine receptors are what triggers preconditioning, then ribosylation of the coupling G proteins with pertussis toxin should block the protective effect of preconditioning.

Rabbits received an intravenous bolus of pertussis toxin, 25 μg/kg, 48 hours prior to the surgical procedure. The potency of the block was tested in each animal with a 0.3 mg/kg iv bolus of acetylcholine. Muscarinic receptors are known to be coupled with inhibitory G protein, G_i, which is pertussis toxin-sensitive. Nontreated animals experienced a 75% decrease in heart rate and a 50% decrease in mean arterial blood pressure. Pertussis toxin limited this acetylcholine effect to only a 10% decrease in heart rate and a 9% decrease in blood pressure. These results indicate that we had significantly, but not completely, blocked G_i with this dose of pertussis toxin.

Pertussis toxin had no effect on infarct size in the nonpreconditioned hearts (infarct size was 37% of the risk zone, which was not different from the 37% seen in the nontreated controls). *Pertussis toxin pretreatment did, however, significantly block the protective effect of preconditioning.* In the presence of pertussis toxin, preconditioned hearts had a mean infarct size of 27% of the risk zone, which was not significantly different from any of the nonpreconditioned groups and was significantly higher than that seen in the preconditioned untreated hearts.

An interesting ramification of the G protein coupling of the adenosine receptors is that other receptors coupled with the same G protein could also initiate preconditioning's protection. Indeed, *we found that the M2 muscarinic agonist, carbachol, was as effective as adenosine in triggering protection* [33]. Lasley et al. also found that they could protect the rat heart with carbachol [34]. M2 receptors are known to be coupled with the pertussis toxin-sensitive G protein, G_i. Another possible trigger for this response might be the alpha-adrenergic receptor, which is also coupled by G_i. In fact, at least one study indicates that alpha agonists can induce preconditioning [35].

PROTEIN KINASE C IS INVOLVED IN THE INTRACELLULAR SIGNALLING PATHWAY

Some isoforms of G_i are also known to activate phospholipase C [36], which cleaves phospholipids in the membrane, causing diacylglycerol (DAG) to be formed. The specific pertussis toxin-sensitive G proteins that couple to phospholipase C include G. That differentiates it from G_q, which is not pertussis toxin sensitive [36]. DAG, in turn, activates protein kinase C, which phosphorylates key proteins in the cell. To test for a role of protein kinase C in ischemic preconditioning, we used its inhibitor, staurosporine, in the in situ rabbit infarct model [37]. Injection of 50 μg/kg of staurosporine 5 minutes prior to the 30-minute ischemia completely blocked protection in preconditioned hearts but did not alter infarct size in the control hearts (41% infarction in preconditioned vs. 36% in control). *Thus preconditioning's protection requires kinase activity during the long ischemia.*

We used isolated rabbit hearts for the converse experiment [37]. We infused 0.01 nmole/min 4β-phorbol 12-myristate 13-acetate (PMA), a protein kinase C activator, into the perfusate for 5 minutes. After a 10-minute recovery period, 30 minutes of regional ischemia was induced followed by 2 hours of reperfusion. Infarct size was much smaller (6% of the risk zone) in the PMA-treated group as compared to the controls (28% of the risk zone). The most likely explanation for this observation is that adenosine receptor occupancy in the ischemic myocyte activates protein kinase C, which in turn activates some protein effector, perhaps an ion channel or a cytoskeletal element, by phosphorylating it. Armstrong and Ganote [38] report that okadaic acid, a blocker of the phosphatases that dephosphorylate those proteins (serine/threonine residues), was very protective in their ischemic myocyte model.

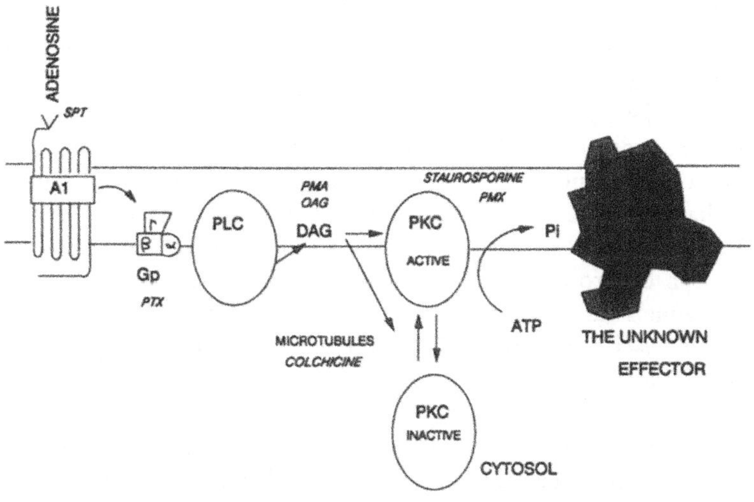

Figure 5. A summary of the intracellular signalling pathways potentially involved in preconditioning in the rabbit. The A_1 adenosine receptor couples to the G protein, G_p, and activates phospholipase C (PLC), which degrades phospholipid in the membrane to diacyl glycerol (DAG). DAG in turn activates protein kinase C (PKC) that is in the membrane and also causes translocation of PKC from the cytosol to the membrane. This translocation is accomplished by microtubules, which can be blocked by colchicine. During ischemia, phosphorylation of an unidentified protein mediates the actual protection. Because translocation is a slow step, taking 5–10 minutes, prior occupation of adenosine receptors during preconditioning allows PKC to be in place from the onset of the long ischemia and thus facilitates early phosphorylation of protein. The words in italics indicate interventions used to test the hypothesis. PTX = pertussis toxin; SPT = 8-p-sulphophenyl theophylline (adenosine receptor blocker); PMA = phorbol 12-myristate 13-acetate; OAG = oleoylacetyl-glycerol; PMX = polymixin B.

How adenosine upregulates the protein kinase C pathway is not known but could be the result of a translocation of protein kinase C into an active compartment such as the membrane. Bogoyevitch et al. [39] report that phorbol esters cause a rapid translocation of protein kinase C epsilon from the cytosol into the membranes of rat myocytes and that it remains in the membranes for about an hour. Thus, activation of phospholipase C by a short period of A_1 receptor occupancy would release DAG, which would first act to translocate protein kinase C into the membrane. Only after the translocation was complete would continued receptor occupancy result in actual kinase activity. We have recently tested this theory by blocking microtubule activity (the process by which protein kinase C is translocated) with colchicine. Pretreating rabbits with 5 mg/kg colchicine completely blocked the protective effect of ischemic preconditioning but had no effect on nonpreconditioned rabbits (unpublished observation).

DOES BLOCKADE OF ATP-SENSITIVE POTASSIUM CHANNELS BLOCK PRECONDITIONING?

While the above studies reveal the involvement of G proteins and a kinase in preconditioning, the effector they are targeted to is less clear. Gross and Auchampach [40] propose that opening of ATP-sensitive potassium channels mediate preconditioning. This is an attractive theory in that Kirsch et al. [41] found that adenosine and A_1-selective analogs opened ATP-sensitive potassium channels in rat ventricular myocytes through activation of G_i protein. Furthermore, several investigators have proposed that opening of potassium channels can be protective to the ischemic heart [42,43]. ATP-sensitive potassium channels can be selectively inhibited by glibenclamide. Indeed, Gross and Auchampach [40] found that glibenclamide did block protection from preconditioning in the dog heart, as did another channel blocker, 6 hydroxydecanoate [44]. Most recently this group was able to block adenosine-induced protection with a potassium channel blocker [45]. It has also been reported that glibenclamide blocks preconditioning in pigs (D.M. Van Winkle, personal communication).

We therefore examined the effect of glibenclamide in our rabbit model of preconditioning. Glibenclamide was given at three different doses (3.0, 0.3, and 0.15 mg/kg), but the preconditioned animals in each of the glibenclamide-treated groups all had significantly smaller infarcts than in the comparable drug-treated controls [46]. Two additional groups were treated with the potassium channel agonist pinacidil at doses of 0.5 and 1.0 mg/kg. This treatment resulted in infarct sizes that were again not significantly different from the untreated controls (32% and 37%, respectively). We were also unable to block preconditioning in the rat heart with glibenclamide [47].

An interesting development in the potassium channel story has recently occurred. The efficacy of glibenclamide in blocking preconditioning seems to depend on the anesthetic agent. We originally used sodium pentobarbital anesthesia for our rabbit study [46]. Toombs et al. [48], using ketamine-xylazine anesthetized rabbits, recently reported that U-89232, an opener of the ATP-dependent potassium channel, did limit infarct size. They also have found (personal communication) that glibenclamide at the 0.3 mg/kg dose selectively blocked preconditioning's protection. We recently examined a series of rabbits anesthetized with ketamine xylazine and confirmed the Toombs et al. observation (data as yet unpublished). *Why the anesthetic agent affects the ability of glibenclamide to block preconditioning remains a mystery, but these data raise doubts about whether the ATP-sensitive potassium channel is the final effector of protection.* It might be that ATP-sensitive potassium channels, in combination with the anesthetic agent, affect the interstitial adenosine levels during ischemia, but this theory remains to be proven.

ADENOSINE DOES NOT APPEAR TO BE INVOLVED IN PRECONDITIONING IN THE RAT

While the story appears convincing that adenosine is important in preconditioning in the rabbit [22,22], the dog [28], and the pig [49], we have been unable to show a similar role in the rat. Rats do exhibit an antiinfarct effect when preconditioned [3,50], which is very similar in magnitude to that seen in rabbits. We were unable to block preconditioning in rats with either PD 115,199 [47] or with pertussis toxin [51]. Preliminary unpublished studies from our laboratory indicate that staurosporine also cannot block preconditioning in rats. These results are discouraging because the protective effect of preconditioning in the rat heart appears too similar to that in other species to not share a common mechanism. While A_1 agonists are protective to the rat heart [9,34,47], adenosine is simply not the trigger for ischemic preconditioning. It is hoped that the reason for this fundamental difference can eventually be resolved.

One further word of caution should be said about the rat model. Preconditioning protocols in the *isolated* rat heart are very effective at preserving postischemic function, and this model is currently in wide use [52–54]. Whether the effect of preconditioning on preserving postischemic function is one and the same as occurs with its antiinfarct effect is currently unknown. In fact, preconditioning definitely does not preserve postischemic function in the in vivo canine model [55], and we have been unable to see this effect in isolated rabbit hearts (unpublished observation) but have seen it in the in situ rabbit heart [56]. Care should be taken when extrapolating data among the models. The same can be said about preconditioning's antiarrhythmic effect [5–7]. For example, we found that one 5-minute ischemia provided protection against subsequent ischemia-induced arrhythmias in the rat heart, but three 5-minute episodes of ischemia were required to achieve an antiinfarct effect [47]. One obvious explanation is that the antiinfarct and the antiarrhythmic effects may involve two separate mechanisms.

CONCLUDING REMARKS

The studies cited above make a strong case for adenosine being a potent antiinfarction agent when given exogenously. In addition, the heart is apparently able to capitalize on this protective property of adenosine and employ it in the preconditioning phenomenon. While we have been able to shed some light on the receptor subtype and the intracellular signalling pathways, the overall mechanism of how A_1 receptor occupancy protects the ischemic heart remains unknown. We have examined the endogenous antioxidants in preconditioned myocardium and found no differences [57]. In addition, as reviewed in Chapter 6, protein synthesis inhibitors fail to block the protective effect of preconditioning, making synthesis of a protective protein an unlikely mechanism [2].

Whether adenosine or A_1-selective analogs can be utilized to protect the patient with acute myocardial infarction remains to be seen. Authentic adenosine would probably have to be selectively infused into the coronary artery to precondition patients, as iv injection would cause too many deleterious side effects at the doses required. Furthermore, mounting evidence indicates that adenosine is also the mediator of the sensation of anginal pain, introducing yet another negative side effect [58]. The requirement for pretreatment and intracoronary administration makes adenosine itself an unlikely clinical choice for patients with acute myocardial infarction, but both of those requirements could be met in the surgical setting.

Our experience with the A_1-selective analogs offers more promise, but their side effects, which include hypotension, bradycardia, narcosis, bronchial spasm, and renal arterial constriction, still appear to be overwhelming. We may have to wait until the final intracellular effector for the adenosine receptor can be identified until we can design a safe and efficient drug that confers preconditioning's protection. In the meantime, adenosine can certainly be a useful tool to aid in identifying that effector.

REFERENCES

1. Murry CE, Jennings RB, Reimer KA. 1986. Preconditioning with ischemia: A delay of lethal cell injury in ischemic myocardium. Circulation 74:1124–1136.
2. Thornton J, Striplin S, Liu GS, Swafford A, Stanley AWH, Van Winkle DM, Downey JM. 1990. Inhibition of protein synthesis does not block myocardial protection afforded by preconditioning. Am J Physiol 259:H1822–H1825.
3. Li Y, Whittaker P, Kloner RA. 1992. The transient nature of the effect of ischemic preconditioning on myocardial infarct size and ventricular arrhythmia. Am Heart J 123:346–353.
4. Schott RJ, Rohmann S, Braun ER, Schaper W. 1990. Ischemic preconditioning reduces infarct size in swine myocardium. Circ Res 66:1133–1142.
5. Shiki K, Hearse DJ. 1987. Preconditioning of ischemic myocardium: Reperfusion-induced arrhythmias. Am J Physiol 253:H1470–H1476.
6. Hagar JM, Hale SL, Kloner RA. 1991. Effect of preconditioning ischemia on reperfusion arrhythmias after coronary artery occlusion and reperfusion in the rat. Circ Res 68:61–68.
7. Vegh A, Sekeres L, Parratt JR. 1990. Protective effects of preconditioning of the ischaemic myocardium involve cyclo-oxygenase products. Cardiovasc Res 24:1020–1023.
8. Belardinelli L, Linden J, Berne R. 1989. The cardiac effects of adenosine. Prog Cardiovasc Dis 32:73–97.
9. Ely SW, Mentzer RM, Jr., Lasley RD, Lee BK, Berne RM. 1985. Functional and metabolic evidence of enhanced myocardial tolerance to ischemia and reperfusion with adenosine. J Thorac Cardiovasc Surg 90:549–556.
10. Van Winkle DM, Thornton JD, Downey DM, Downey JM. 1991. The natural history of preconditioning: Cardioprotection depends on duration of transient ischemia and time to subsequent ischemia. Coronary Artery Dis 2:613–619.
11. Li GC, Vasquez JA, Gallagher KP, Lucchesi BR. 1990. Myocardial protection with preconditioning. Circulation 82:609–619.
12. Van Wylen DG, Willis J, Sodhi J, Weiss R, Lasley RD, Mentzer RM. 1990. Cardiac microdialysis to estimate interstitial adenosine and coronary blood flow. Am J Physiol 258:H1642–H1649.
13. Iwamoto T, Miura T, Adachi T, Noto T, Ogawa T, Tsuchida A, II, Iimura O. 1991. Myocardial infarct size-limiting effect of ischemic preconditioning was not attenuated by oxygen free-radical scavengers in the rabbit. Circulation 83:1015–1022.

14. Miura T, Yellon DM, Hearse DJ, Downey JM. 1987. Determinants of infarct size during permanent occlusion of a coronary artery in the closed chest dog. J Am Coll Cardiol 9:647–654.
15. Reimer KA, Jennings RB. 1979. The wavefront phenomenon of myocardial ischemic cell death. II. Transmural progression of necrosis within the framework of ischemic bed size (myocardium at risk) and collateral flow. Lab Invest 40:633–640.
16. Liu GS, Thornton J, Van Winkle DM, Stanley AWH, Olsson RA, Downey JM. 1991. Protection against infarction afforded by preconditioning is mediated by A1 adenosine receptors in rabbit heart. Circulation 84:350–356.
17. Van Winkle DM, Chien GL, Wolff RA, Soifer BE, David RF. 1992. Intracoronary infusion of R-phenylisopropyl adenosine prior to ischemia/reperfusion reduces myocardial infarct size in swine. Circulation 86(Suppl I):I213 (abstr).
18. Grover GJ, Sleph PG, Dzwonczyk S, Sargent CA. 1992. Role of ATP-sensitive potassium channels (KATP) in preconditioning in the dog heart and their interaction with adenosine A1 receptors. Circulation 86(Suppl I):I341 (abstr).
19. Toombs CF, McGee DS, Johnston WE, Vinten-Johansen J. 1992. Myocardial protective effects of adenosine: Infarct size reduction with pretreatment and continued receptor stimulation during ischemia. Circulation 86:986–994.
20. Lohse MJ, Klotz KN, Schwabe U, Cristalli G, Vittori S, Grifantini M. 1988. 2-Chloro-N-cyclopentyladenosine: A highly selective agonist at A1 adenosine receptors. Naunyn-Schmiedebergs Arch Pharmacol 337:687–689.
21. Tsuchida A, Liu G, Downey J. 1992. Pretreatment with adenosine A1 selective agonist CCPA limits infarct size in a chronic rabbit model. Circulation 86(Suppl I):I23 (abstr).
22. Tsuchida A, Miura T, Miki T, Shimamoto K, Iimura O. 1992. Role of adenosine receptor activation in myocardial infarct size limitation by ischemic preconditioning. Cardiovasc Res 26:456–461.
23. Thornton JD, Liu GS, Olsson RA, Downey JM. 1992. Intravenous pretreatment with A1-selective adenosine analogues protects the heart against infarction. Circulation 85:659–665.
24. Tsuchida A, Liu GS, Mullane K, Downey JM. 1993. Acadesine lowers the temporal threshold for the myocardioal infarct size limiting effect of preconditioning. Cardiovasc Res, in press.
25. Miura T, Ogawa T, Iwamoto T, Shimamoto K, Iimura O. 1992. Dipyridamole potentiates the myocardial infarct size-limiting effect of preconditioning. Circulation 86:979–985.
26. Itoya M, Miura T, Urabe K. 1992. Nucleoside transport inhibitors enhance the infarct size limiting effect of preconditioning. Circulation 86(Suppl I):I25 (abstr).
27. Thornton J, Downey J. 1992. Blocking adenosine receptors between preconditioning and prolonged ischemia prevents protection. Circulation 86(Suppl I):I343 (abstr).
28. Kitakaze M, Hori M, Takashima S, Sato H, Inoue M, Kamada T. 1993. Ischemic preconditioning increases adenosine release and 5′ nucleotidase activity during myocardial ischemia and reperfusion in dogs: Implications for myocardial salvage. Circulation 87:208–215.
29. Kitakaze M, Kitabatake A. 1991. Increased 5′ nucleotidase activity caused by protein kinase C enhances adenosine production in hypoxic cardiomyocytes. Circulation 84(Suppl II):II620 (abstr).
30. Tsuchida A, Olsson RA, Downey JM. 1993. Cardioprotective effect of CCPA is lost after 72 hour infusion along with the ability to precondition. FASEB J 7, in press.
31. Brown AM. 1990. Regulation of heartbeat by G protein-coupled ion channels. Am J Physiol 259:H1621–H1628.
32. Stiles GL. 1991. Adenosine receptors: Physiologic regulation and biochemical mechanisms. NIPS 6:161–165.
33. Thornton JD, Downey JM. 1992. Pretreatment with pertussis toxin blocks the protective effects of preconditioning: Evidence for a Gi-protein mechanism. J Mol Cell Cardiol, in press.
34. Lasley RD, Van Wylen DGL, Mentzer RM. 1990. Evidence for the role of Gi proteins in attenuating myocardial ischemic damage. Circulation 82(Suppl III):III759 (abstr).
35. Locke-Winter C, Winter C, Nelson D, Banerjee A. 1991. cAMP stimulation facilitates preconditioning against ischemia-reperfusion through norepinephrine and $alpha_1$ mechanism. Circulation 84(Suppl II):II1722 (abstr).

36. Fleming JW, Wisler PL, Watanabe AM. 1992. Signal transduction by G proteins in cardiac tissues. Circulation 85:419–433.
37. Ytrehus K, Liu Y, Downey JM. 1993. Preconditioning protects the ischemic rabbit heart by protein kinase activation. FASEB J, in press.
38. Armstrong SC, Ganote CE. 1992. Effects of protein phosphatase inhibitors okadaic acid and calyculin A on metabolically inhibited and ischaemic isolated myocytes. J Mol Cell Cardiol 24:869–884.
39. Bogoyevitch MA, Parker PJ, Sugden PH. 1993. Characterization of protein kinase C expression in adult rat heart. Circ Res 72:757–767.
40. Gross GJ, Auchampach JA. 1992. Blockade of ATP-sensitive potassium channels prevents myocardial preconditioning in dogs. Circ Res 70:223–233.
41. Kirsch GE, Codina J, Birnbaumer L, Brown AM. 1990. Coupling of ATP-sensitive K^+ channels to A1 receptors by G proteins in rat ventricular myocytes. Am J Physiol 259:-H820–H826.
42. Cole WC, McPherson CD, Sontag D. 1991. ATP-regulated K + channels protect the myocardium against ischemia/reperfusion damage. Circ Res 69:571–581.
43. Grover G, Sleph P, Dzwonczyk S. 1990. Reduction of ischemic/reperfusion damage in isolated rat hearts by the potassium channel opener RP 52891. J Mol Cell Cardiol 22(Suppl III):S.6 (abstr).
44. Auchampach JA, Gross GJ. 1992. Blockade of ischaemic preconditioning in dogs by the novel ATP dependent potassium channel antagonist sodium 5-hydroxydecanoate. Cardiovasc Res 26:1054–1062.
45. Auchampach JA, Gross GJ. 1992. Activation of ATP-dependent potassium (K_{ATP}) channels by adenosine: A possible mechanism for ischemic preconditioning in dogs. Circulation 86(Suppl I):I345 (abstr).
46. Thornton J, Thornton CS, Sterling DL, Downey JM. 1993. Blockade of ATP-sensitive potassium channels increases infarct size but does not prevent preconditioning in rabbit hearts. Circ Res 72:44–49.
47. Liu Y, Downey JM. 1992. Ischemic preconditioning protects against infarction in rat heart. Am J Physiol 263:H1107–H1112.
48. Toombs CF, Norman NR, Shebuski RJ. 1992. Reduction of infarct size with U-89232: A non-vasoactive analog of the potassium channel opener chromakalim. Circulation 86(Suppl I):I556 (abstr).
49. Schwarz ER, Mohri M, Sack S, Arras M. 1991. The role of adenosine and its A1-receptor in ischemic preconditioning. Circulation 84(Suppl II):II191 (abstr).
50. Li Y, Kloner RA. 1992. Is ischemic "preconditioning" mediated by cardioprotective prostanoids?. Cardiovasc Res 26:226–231.
51. Liu Y, Downey JM. 1993. Preconditioning against infarction in the rat heart does not involve a pertussis toxin-sensitive G protein. Cardiovasc Res, in press.
52. Asimakis G, Inners-McBride K, Medellin G, Conti V. 1992. Ischemic preconditioning attenuates acidosis and postischemic dysfunction in the isolated rat heart. Am J Physiol 263:H887–H894.
53. Cave AC, Downey JM, Hearse DJ. 1991. Adenosine fails to substitute for preconditioning in the globally ischemic isolated rat heart. J Mol Cell Cardiol 23(Suppl III):S76 (abstr).
54. Locke-Winter CR, Winter CB, Nelson DW, Banerjee A. 1991. cAMP stimulation facilitates preconditioning against ischemia-reperfusion through norepinephrine and $alpha_1$ mechanism. Circulation 84(Suppl II):II433 (abstr).
55. Ovize M, Przyklenk K, Hale SL, Kloner RA. 1992. Preconditioning does not attenuate myocardial stunning. Circulation 85:2247–2254.
56. Cohen MV, Liu GS, Downey JM. 1991. Preconditioning causes improved wall motion as well as smaller infarcts after transient coronary occlusion in rabbits. Circulation 84:341–349.
57. Turrens JF, Thornton J, Barnard ML, Snyder S, Liu G, Downey JM. 1992. Protection from reperfusion injury by preconditioning hearts does not involve increased antioxidant defenses. Am J Physiol 262:H585–H589.
58. Crea F, Pupita G, Galassi AR, El-Tamimi H, Kaski JC, Davies G, Maseri A. 1990. Role of adenosine in pathogenesis of anginal pain. Circulation 81:164–172.

9. SYNOPSIS OF ISCHEMIC PRECONDITIONING: WHAT HAVE WE LEARNED SINCE 1986?

KARIN PRZYKLENK, ROBERT A. KLONER, and PETER WHITTAKER

CHARACTERISTICS OF PRECONDITIONING: THE GOOD, THE INDIFFERENT—AND THE BAD? (TABLE 1)

Reduction in infarct size

There is no question that preconditioning with brief ischemia acutely delays myocyte death and thereby limits infarct size. *As reviewed by Murry and colleagues in Chapter 1, this reduction in infarct size has, since their initial report in 1986, been a consistent finding among all laboratories and in every model and species in which this concept has been evaluated.* Such unanimous agreement among laboratories is indeed a rare event in the study of myocardial ischemia and infarction! In addition, as described by Reimer et al. in Chapter 5, there is little doubt that the reduction in infarct size with preconditioning is associated with a slowing in the rate of myocardial energy metabolism during the initial phase of the subsequent sustained coronary occlusion. Importantly, however, we have also come to recognize the temporal limitations of this cardioprotective phenomenon. Evidence from several models indicates that *the protective effect is transient*: While the specific time constraints vary somewhat among species, the sustained occlusion must, in the dog model, (1) be limited to less than 90 minutes and (2) follow soon (i.e., on the order of 1–2 hours) after the brief ischemia.

Table 1. Characteristics of preconditioning

Beneficial effect on	Current evidence	Comments
Infarct size/cell viability?	Yes	Delay of cell death confirmed in all species and models studied to date
Rate of energy utilization during the early phase of sustained ischemia?	Yes	
In vivo contractile function of viable but "stunned" myocardium?	Acute: No	Improved function in some acute studies due to reduction in infarct size/preservation of cell viability?
	Chronic: ?	Effect of preconditioning on *rate of recovery* of function remains unknown.
Arrhythmias?	Inconclusive	Yes in the rat model; but uncertain in other species
Coronary vasculature?	Inconclusive	
Myocardial collagen?	No (?)	Indirect evidence demonstrates that repeated brief ischemia *damages*, rather than protects, myocardial collagen

Other sequelae of ischemia/reperfusion

The stunned myocardium

In contrast to the consensus among studies that preconditioning limits infarct size, the effects of ischemic preconditioning on other deleterious sequelae of sustained occlusion/reperfusion are less well defined. For example, as reviewed by Ovize et al., in Chapter 3, studies to date performed in isolated globally ischemic heart preparations have consistently reported improved recovery of left ventricular developed pressure in hearts "preconditioned" with brief episodes of antecedent global ischemia. The important question is: Is this improved contractile function a secondary consequence of a reduction in cellular necrosis, or do these data indicate that preconditioning enhances recovery of function of viable but "stunned" myocytes? In the isolated heart model, this question remains unanswered. However, evidence from the in vivo canine model indicates that preconditioning does not result in an acute improvement in wall motion of the stunned myocardium during the initial hours following reflow [2]. Whether preconditioning accelerates the recovery of function of stunned myocardium during the days to weeks following relief of ischemia has not, to date, been investigated.

Arrhythmias

Considerable investigative effort has also focused on the effects of preconditioning on ischemia- and reperfusion-induced arrhythmias. As described by Lawson and Hearse in Chapter 2, the substantial body of work done in the rat model leaves no doubt that, in this species, ischemic preconditioning markedly attenuates the incidence of ventricular tachycardia, fibrillation, and premature beats. Moreover, this protection against arrhythmias is "dose-dependent"; i.e., there is greater protection with multiple episodes of preconditioning ischemia than with one brief ischemic insult [3]. However, in contrast to the consistent finding of infarct size reduction among all species studied, the effects of preconditioning on arrhythmias in the dog, rabbit, and swine models is uncertain. The lack of an obvious antiarrhythmic effect in these other models may, as suggested by Lawson and Hearse, simply reflect the fact that most studies using dogs, rabbits, and pigs were not designed to assess arrhythmias as a primary end point. Thus, it remains unclear whether preconditioning attenuates ventricular arrhythmias in all models, or whether this facet of protection is unique to the rat.

Deterioration in resting myocardial perfusion and loss of coronary vasodilator reserve

Do the benefits of ischemic preconditioning extend beyond the myocyte and include the coronary vasculature? To date, only three studies have addressed this issue and, as detailed by Bauer et al. in Chapter 4, the results have been mixed. One report has found that in the anesthetized open-chest dog, preconditioning preserves both serotonin- and acetylcholine-mediated increases in coronary arteriolar diameter [4]. However, in a similar canine model, our laboratory has found that brief preconditioning ischemia: (1) failed to prevent "low reflow" (i.e., the deterioration in resting blood flow to viable myocardium following relief of ischemia); and (2) failed to attenuate the loss in endothelium-dependent and endothelium-independent vasodilator reserve (i.e., the increase in coronary blood flow in response to acetylcholine and nitroglycerin challenge, respectively), which occurs following relief of sustained coronary occlusion [5]. The reason for this apparent discrepancy between studies is unknown.

Damage to the collagen matrix: Myocardial "deconditioning"? (Figure 1)

One issue that to date, has not been directly addressed in these various protocols is the effect of preconditioning on the collagen matrix of the heart. This concept may be of importance, as at least two studies have provided disturbing evidence that multiple brief episodes of coronary occlusion — without subsequent sustained occlusion — can cause collagen damage, even in the absence of myocyte necrosis. Specifically, both our laboratory [6] and others [7] have examined the effect of 12 repeated 5-minute coronary artery occlusions, each separated by 10 minutes of reperfusion, on regional myocardial contractile function and the structural integrity of the collagen fibroskeleton in canine myocardium. Scanning electron microscopy revealed areas of the myocardium that appeared totally devoid of collagen and, in other areas, evidence of broken and disrupted collagen fibrils [7]. Although this apparent complete loss of collagen in localized areas was, in our hands, not confirmed by light microscopy, we did observe what appeared to be

A

B

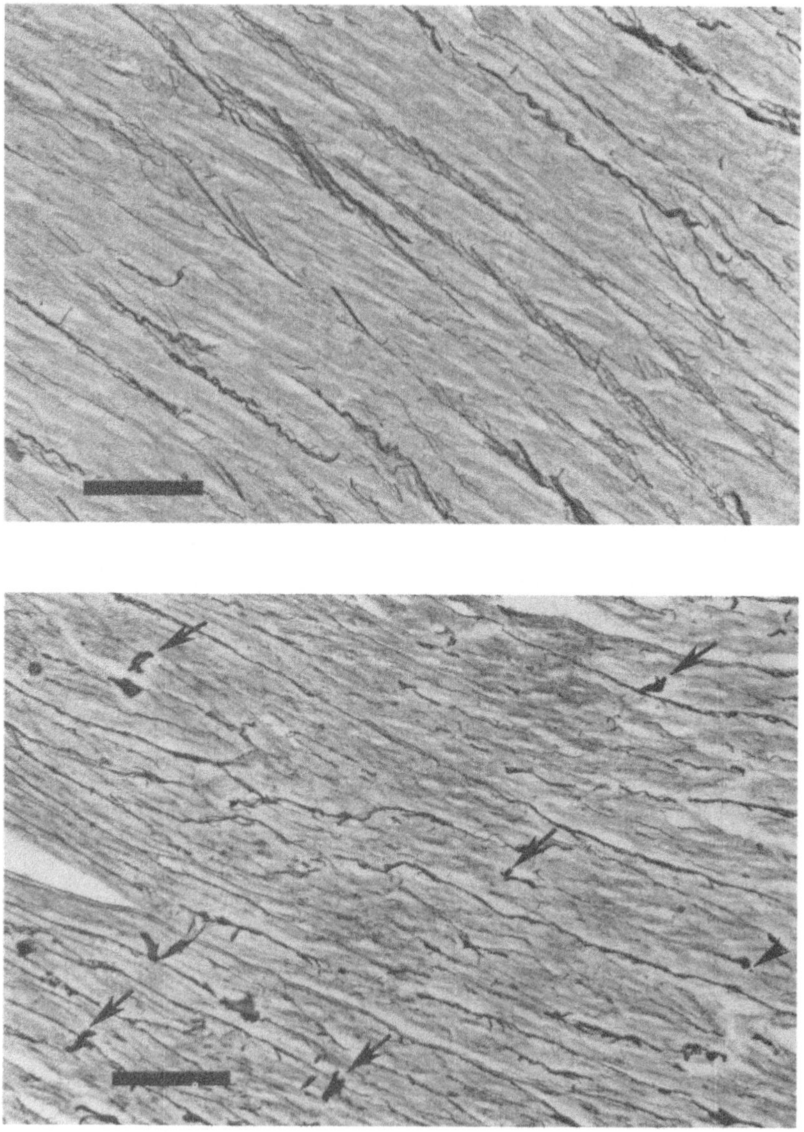

Figure 1. Micrographs of silver-impregnated histologic sections obtained from (**A**) nonischemic control myocardium and (**B**) myocardium subjected to 12 episodes of (15 minutes ischemia + 5 minutes reperfusion). Collagen fiber strands, stained grey-black by this technique, appear shorter and darker in the tissue subjected to repeated ischemia, suggesting the presence of broken fibers (highlighted by the arrows) and a difference in the binding of silver particles to the collagen. Furthermore, when the sections were viewed with polarized light, there was a reduction in the birefringence or brightness of collagen fibers in tissue subjected to repeated ischemia, even though the myocytes retained their birefringence; that is, there was evidence of collagen damage in the absence of muscle necrosis following repeated brief ischemia. Bar = 50 μm.

broken collagen fibers in the ischemic/reperfused tissue [6]. In addition, we saw a marked reduction in the brightness or birefringence of silver-impregnated collagen fibers viewed by polarized light microscopy and, as silver is thought to attach to the ground substance associated with the collagen, we speculated that the observed loss of birefringence indicated damage to the ground substance [6]. We do not know the mechanism responsible for this collagen injury, although the heart is known to contain collagenase, which may somehow be activated by the repeated occlusion.

It should be noted that (1) both studies focused exclusively on the acute phase of ischemia/reperfusion, and (2) both studies in essence involved a "preconditioning regimen" *without* an additional period of sustained ischemia. The first point may be important, as we do not know the long-term consequences of collagen damage induced by brief ischemia. Does the collagen matrix return to its original organization, is it lost forever, or does the injury stimulate the formation of significant fibrosis? The issue of the lack of a sustained period of ischemia in the two studies could be even more important, as longer periods of ischemia have also been shown to result in collagen damage. For example, in the rat model, evidence from our laboratory indicates that the amount of collagen damage increases with time after permanent coronary artery occlusion, and that the degree of collagen damage is a crucial mediator of deleterious topographic changes such as infarct expansion [8]. Thus, despite the reduction in infarct size achieved by preconditioning, collagen damage due to repeated preconditioning ischemia, if added to that produced by prolonged ischemia, could conceivably exacerbate infarct expansion. We are currently examining such possibilities.

It has been shown that even a single brief episode of coronary occlusion can protect the heart against subsequent sustained ischemia, and, in fact, most studies to date have used one to four episodes of preconditioning ischemia. It could therefore be argued that the finding of collagen damage after 12 periods of brief ischemia is of little relevance. However, two points should be considered. First, if we foster the hope that angina might trigger a cardioprotective response analogous to preconditioning in patients with coronary artery disease (a concept addressed in Chapter 10), such episodes rarely occur as single or isolated events; that is, preconditioning by angina may be more closely approximated by the 12 occlusion model, rather than the one to four occlusions that are usually used experimentally. Secondly, if the temporal constraints of preconditioning described in Chapter 1 hold true clinically, then in instances of extended delay between angina and sustained ischemia or extended duration of coronary occlusion, the collagen damage caused by repeated brief ischemia may exacerbate that caused by sustained ischemia in the absence of any muscle protection.

Thus, although ischemic preconditioning can protect myocytes from a subsequent sustained coronary occlusion, repeated brief ischemia may also cause profound injury to the myocardial connective tissue matrix. How such collagen injury occurs, how many brief occlusions are necessary to produce collagen injury, and the ultimate consequences of this collagen damage are all unknown. Nevertheless, indirect evidence suggests that, under certain circumstances, repeated brief periods of ischemia may damage or "decondition" the myocardial collagen matrix while protecting or "preconditioning" the myocytes. This issue, we believe, warrants further evaluation.

MECHANISM(S) OF INFARCT SIZE REDUCTION BY PRECONDITIONING: CURRENT THINKING (TABLE 2 AND FIGURE 2)

While there is no doubt that ischemic preconditioning can limit infarct size, the question of *why* brief ischemia should be cardioprotective is unresolved. Not surprising, there has been no shortage of theories put forward to explain this phenomenon.

Preconditioning is not explained by an increase in collateral perfusion

The first and most obvious explanation for the reduction in infarct size with preconditioning is that brief episodes of coronary occlusion might act as a stimulus to "open" collateral channels and thereby attenuate the severity of the subsequent sustained ischemia. This is, at least in the dog model, not the case: Repeated measurements of regional myocardial blood flow have revealed no increase in collateral perfusion during the brief vs. prolonged ischemic episodes [9]. Interestingly, however, a trend toward an increase in blood flow to the ischemic myocardium has been observed in preconditioned

Table 2. Mechanism(s) of infarct size reduction by preconditioning

Mechanism	Current evidence	Comments
Increase in collateral blood flow?	No	Conclusive in the dog and pig models, but may play a role in the rabbit?
Synthesis of protective protein?	No	Cannot explain acute protection, but may provide a "second window" of protection
Paradoxical protection by oxygen radicals/enhanced production of antioxidants?	Unlikely	Questionable whether the time course of enhanced antioxidant production would be compatible with acute protection
Inhibition of mitochondrial ATPase?	No	Rats can be preconditioned, despite an absence of the ATPase inhibitor
Activation of the adenosine A_1 receptor?	Inconclusive	Supported in the rabbit model, but inconclusive in other species
Opening of the K_{ATP} channel?	Inconclusive	Supported in the dog and pig, but not confirmed in other species
Antiadrenergic mechanism?	Inconclusive	Only evidence to date is from preliminary reports in the isolated rat heart

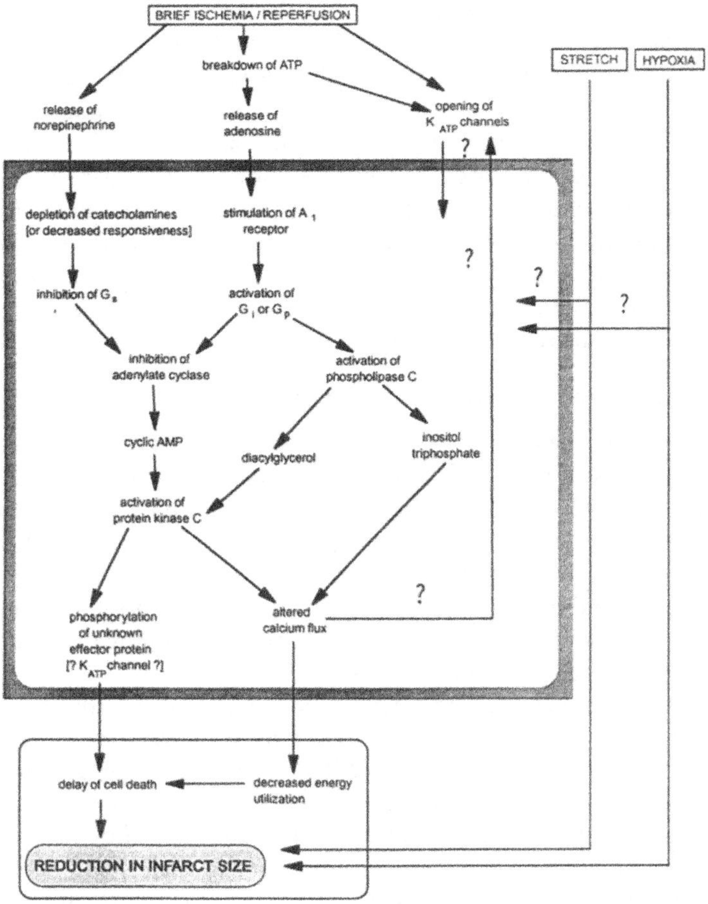

Figure 2. Summary of current theories thought to explain cardioprotection by brief periods of ischemia/reperfusion. Although the components of the secondary messenger pathways (enclosed in this stippled border) have been well characterized [25,26], the role of these pathways as the intermediary between brief ischemia/reperfusion and reduction in infarct size remains the subject of ongoing investigation. Whether the protective effects of other stimuli such as stretch and/or hypoxia are mediated by the same mechanism(s) as brief ischemia/reperfusion is unknown.

rabbits between 2.5 and 35 minutes of sustained coronary occlusion [10]. The implications of this observation have not, however, been pursued in subsequent studies of preconditioning that have used the rabbit model.

Acute protection is not due to synthesis of a protective protein

A more novel hypothesis to explain infarct size reduction by preconditioning is that brief ischemia might trigger the synthesis of a protective protein, such as heat shock protein (hsp), and thereby protect the heart from a subsequent more sustained ischemic insult. Production of hsp is, in fact, triggered in the myocardium by brief ischemia [11], and there is no doubt that these proteins are cardioprotective [12,13]. However, as reviewed by Marber, Heads, and Yellon in Chapter 6, the time course of the synthesis of these proteins (on the order of hours) is not compatible with the acute reduction in infarct size seen with ischemic preconditioning, where the sustained occlusion is initiated within minutes of the brief ischemia. Although the synthesis of protective proteins cannot explain the acute reduction in infarct size that is the hallmark of preconditioning, there is evidence to suggest that protective proteins induced by brief ischemia may provide a "second window of protection" 24 hours later [14]. However, very recent data indicate that even this delayed protection may prove to be transient [15].

Oxygen radicals and antioxidant enzymes

Oxygen-derived radicals have been the focus of considerable investigative effort during the past decade, in that these compounds have been implicated to play a role in lethal "reperfusion injury" [16]. But despite their cytotoxic properties, it has been suggested that oxygen radicals generated during brief episodes of ischemia/reperfusion may paradoxically protect the heart from subsequent sustained ischemia, and/or brief preconditioning ischemia may enhance the production of endogenous antioxidant or free radical scavengers and thereby provide cardioprotection.

The issue of paradoxical protection by oxygen radicals has been addressed by administration of exogenous free radical scavenging agents (such as superoxide dismutase + catalase [17] and N-2-mercaptopropionyl glycine [18]) during the preconditioning regimen. The entire spectrum of possible outcomes has been obtained: Some investigators have shown that free radical scavengers attenuated the reduction in infarct size with preconditioning [18], other groups have reported no effect [17,19], while others have found intermediate results (i.e., preconditioning was abolished in some animals but not in others) [20]. These inconsistencies may be a consequence of the problems that have plagued the use of free radical scavengers throughout the past decade in the study of reperfusion injury: What dose should be used? How can sufficient quantities of these agents be delivered into a region of severely ischemic myocardium receiving negligible blood flow? Do the scavenging agents cross the cell membrane? These fundamental questions remain unanswered.

Does preconditioning trigger the enhanced production of endogenous antioxidants and free radical scavenging agents? Once again the data are inconclusive: Both positive [21] and negative results [22] have been obtained. But, as was the case with heat shock proteins, it is questionable whether the time course of an increased synthesis or release of antioxidant or scavenging enzymes would be compatible with the acute time course of the preconditioning phenomenon.

The adenosine hypothesis

Downey and colleagues sparked the interest of investigators in 1991 by providing evidence that activation of the adenosine A_1 receptor, presumably by adenosine released during the brief preconditioning ischemia, was a pivotal mediator of the reduction in infarct size seen in preconditioned animals vs. controls [23,24]. Through the use of a host of agonists and antagonists acting at various loci on well-described secondary messenger pathways [25,26], Downey and coworkers have expanded upon this initial observation and proposed that stimulation of the A_1 receptor triggers a cascade of events that, in brief, involves activation of an inhibitory guanine nucleotide regulatory (G) protein; activation of protein kinase C by diacylglycerol; and, ultimately, limitation of infarct size by the resultant phosphorylation of an as yet-unidentified effector protein. The details of this pathway are described by Downey et al. in Chapter 8 and are illustrated in Figure 2.

One important factor in the consideration of the adenosine hypothesis is that virtually all of the firm evidence in support of this concept has been obtained using the rabbit model. Data from the dog [27,28] and swine models [29,30] is limited, while in the rat, intravenous infusion of adenosine and the use of adenosine agonists and antagonists has proven ineffective in modulating infarct size reduction by preconditioning [31,32]. Thus, despite supportive evidence in the rabbit, the adenosine hypothesis does not, based on the currently available data, appear to provide a "universal" explanation for infarct size reduction with preconditioning.

Opening of ATP-sensitive potassium channels

Gross and Auchampach [33] were the first to report that manipulation of the ATP-sensitive potassium (K_{ATP}) channel by selective agonists and antagonists effectively blunts and mimics infarct size reduction by preconditioning in the dog model. However, as discussed by Gross et al. in Chapter 7, precisely *how* these channels are opened, and *why* this should be cardioprotective, is unknown. It would appear, however, that the K_{ATP} hypothesis and the adenosine hypothesis are closely integrated: There is evidence (albeit limited) that adenosine opens the K_{ATP} channel via an inhibitory G_i protein [34] and that activation of protein kinase C may also open the channel [26]. But, as was the case with the adenosine hypothesis, the role of the K_{ATP} channel in ischemic preconditioning has not been confirmed in all species: While the K_{ATP} channel appears to be important in both the dog [28,33] and pig models [35], data obtained in the rabbit have been inconclusive [36,37] and results in the rat have been negative [32,38].

An "antiadrenergic" mechanism?

One theory that has provoked the curiosity of investigators is that preconditioning may be mediated by an "antiadrenergic" mechanism [39]. Specifically, release of norepinephrine from cardiac nerve terminals during the first brief occlusion (a response that *increases* myocardial energy demand) may attenuate the release of norepinephrine during the subsequent ischemia (perhaps by depletion of norepinephrine stores) and/or result in a decreased responsiveness to subsequent norepinephrine release. Either scenario would result in reduced activation of the stimulatory G_s protein; this, in turn, would presumably activate protein kinase (in this case via cyclic AMP) and, as was the case with the adenosine hypothesis, might ultimately limit infarct size by phosphorylation of an unknown effector protein. Clearly this is not a unique hypothesis, but rather represents an additional point of entry into the secondary messenger pathways (Figure 2).

There is, to date, only preliminary information indicating that in the isolated rat heart, preconditioning (defined as the enhanced recovery of left ventricular pressure following sustained global ischemia) can be attenuated by administration of an alpha-receptor blocker [39]. Whether manipulation of alpha and beta receptors can mediate infarct size reduction and decreased energy demand in other species and models is unknown but, as detailed by Reimer and colleagues in Chapter 5, studies aimed at testing this concept are underway in several laboratories.

Infarct size reduction via altered energy metabolism

Reimer and colleagues have demonstrated that preconditioning attenuates the rate of myocardial energy utilization: As described in detail in Chapter 5, depletion of high energy phosphates and production of lactate are significantly slowed during the initial 20 minutes of sustained coronary occlusion in preconditioned dogs vs. controls [9]. This transient slowing in the rate of energy depletion has emerged as a fundamental concept of the preconditioning phenomenon and, as a result, it has been suggested that any hypothesis for the reduction in infarct size with ischemic preconditioning must also incorporate this observation.

One initially attractive theory to explain the reduction in energy utilization focused on the "wasting" of high energy phosphates during ischemia by hydrolysis of ATP via the enzyme mitochondrial ATPase [40]. Specifically, preconditioning might activate inhibitors of mitochondrial ATPase, thereby reducing energy demand during ischemia and thus limiting infarct size. This theory was seriously challenged by the numerous reports that the rat — a species that lacks the endogenous inhibitor of mitochondrial ATPase — could nonetheless be effectively preconditioned [31,32,41,42]. Vander Heide and colleagues have, in fact, confirmed that inhibition of mitochondrial ATPase is *not* the mechanism responsible for preconditioning [40; see Chapter 5]. This has not, however, disproved the concept that the reduction in infarct size with preconditioning is a consequence of the transient reduction in energy demand: As reviewed by Reimer et al. in Chapter 5, activation of the adenosine A_1 receptor, opening of K_{ATP} channels, and depletion of catecholamines — the current "popular" theories to explain infarct size reduction with preconditioning — may all result in slowing of ATP utilization during sustained ischemia.

CONCEPTUAL QUESTIONS

Is "ischemia" a prerequisite for "ischemic preconditioning"?

"What is the mechanism of ischemic preconditioning?" is only one of the many unanswered questions that has been raised since the initial report of Murry et al. [1]. For example, the use of the term *ischemic* clearly implicates ischemia as an important factor in mediating preconditioning. However, linking the two words may be unnecessarily restrictive, both in terms of our thinking and in the design of experiments to determine the mechanism of protection. A brief transient period of *hypoxia* prior to sustained coronary occlusion has been shown, in the dog model, to reduce infarct size to a similar degree as that produced by a comparable period of brief preconditioning ischemia [43]. Similarly, a transient period of partial coronary *stenosis* in the canine model effectively reduced infarct size produced by a subsequent 1-hour episode of sustained coronary occlusion [44; Figure 2].

Are *hypoxic preconditioning*, *stenotic preconditioning*, and *ischemic preconditioning* all the same phenomenon? The answer to this question is unknown. However, the results obtained using hypoxia and stenosis as the protective stimulus may provide insight into the possible mechanisms of cardioprotection by brief ischemia. For example, hypoxia does not result in the accumulation of interstitial adenosine [43], presumably precluding stimulation of the A_1 receptor as a mechanism of hypoxic preconditioning. With regard to stenotic preconditioning, the protective effects of partial stenosis were only manifest when followed by a period of complete reperfusion prior to sustained coronary occlusion [44]. This suggests that accumulation of metabolites or metabolic adaptation during the period of stenosis was, in itself, insufficient to result in reduction of infarct size, and implies that washout (or perhaps, washin) of substance(s) may be important. The relationship, if any, between hypoxic preconditioning, stenotic preconditioning, and ischemic preconditioning clearly awaits further study.

A "universal" mechanism?

A related question is, if ischemic preconditioning limits infarct size in all models studied, does the same mechanism mediate this phenomenon in all species? Logic would appear to dictate that a common mechanism must be operative but, as summarized in Table 2, no one theory proposed to date has been confirmed in all species. How can we explain the disparate results obtained, for example, with adenosine agonists and antagonists in the rabbit vs. rat models? The apparent discrepancies may mean: (1) the A_1 receptor plays a pivotal role in the rabbit and not in the rat; (2) the A_1 receptor may play a role in both species, but rat and rabbit myocardium may differ in terms of the kinetics of the secondary messenger pathways (i.e., binding affinities of the agonists and antagonists, differences in the rate constants at various steps in the pathway, etc.); or (3) spurious results may, for unknown reasons, have been obtained. The same arguments could be put forward to explain the inconsistences in the K_{ATP} hypothesis: In particular, differences in the choice of anesthetic agents have been implicated as a contributing factor in the differences among protocols (see Chapters 7 and 8). Similarly, logic might suggest that various apparent *consequences* of ischemic preconditioning are due to a common mechanism. However, in the rat model, data from Lawson et al. (summarized in Chapter 2) suggest that reduction in infarct size and attenuation of arrhythmias may be mediated by quite different pathways. Thus, the attractive concept of a universal mechanism may be false and, more importantly, we should not permit this type of preconceived notion to hinder or restrict future research efforts.

Does anesthesia play a role?

Finally, it is interesting to note that all experimental studies of ischemic preconditioning have, to date, involved ischemia/reperfusion in anesthetized in vivo preparations or, in instances of global ischemia, hearts removed following anesthesia. While it appears unlikely that reduction in infarct size by ischemic preconditioning is purely an artifact induced by anesthesia, it is conceivable that the protective effects of ischemic preconditioning may differ to some degree in conscious vs. anesthetized preparations. This is by no means a novel concept; for example, there is some evidence to suggest that the time course and severity of myocardial stunning following brief transient ischemia may differ in pentobarbital-anesthetized vs. conscious dogs [45]. Ischemic preconditioning in a conscious animal model is yet to be characterized.

APPROACHING THE PROBLEM FROM A NEW PERSPECTIVE: A MATHEMATICAL MODEL OF PRECONDITIONING

Theoretical limitations of the agonist/antagonist approach

It is evident from Chapters 5–8 and the preceding discussion that most investigators have turned to cellular biology and focused on well-described secondary messenger pathways in their search to elucidate the mechanism(s) of ischemic preconditioning. As mentioned previously, this has for the most part been approached by the administration of various agonists and antagonists. While this has without question provided valuable insights, interpretation of the results, particularly in in vivo studies, can be confounded by both the profound hemodynamic consequences of many of these agents (i.e., the marked reduction in mean arterial pressure caused by treatment with adenosine and adenosine agonists — see Chapter 8) and the effects of these agents on other organs (i.e., alterations in blood glucose induced by glibenclamide — see Chapter 7). In addition, even if these agents provide defi-

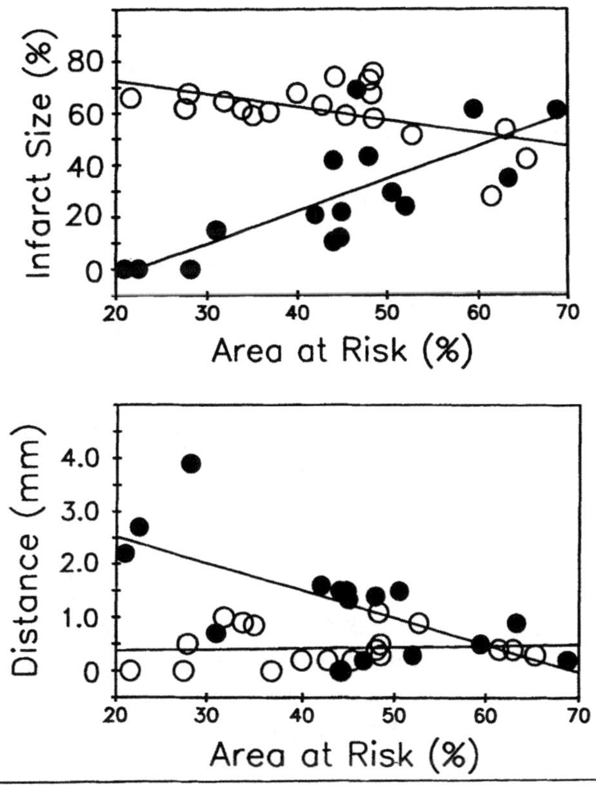

Figure 3. A: Infarct size (expressed as a percent of the area at risk), plotted as a function of the area at risk (expressed as a percent of the total left ventricular weight) for control rats subjected to 90 minutes of sustained coronary occlusion (open circles) and preconditioned rats subjected to three 3-minute episodes of brief ischemia prior to 90 minutes of sustained occlusion (solid circles). In control animals, infarct size was not dependent upon the size of the risk region. In contrast, in preconditioned rats infarct size increased with increasing risk region. **B:** Average lateral distance from the edge of the necrosis to the boundary of the area at risk (expressed as a percent of the total left ventricular weight) for control (open circles) and preconditioned rats (solid circles). The relationship between the extent of lateral salvage and the size of the risk region was significant for the preconditioned rats ($r = 0.67$ and $p = 0.0046$), but not for the controls ($r = 0.08$). Reprinted with permission from Whittaker et al. [47].

nitive information concerning the mechanism of preconditioning, these unfavorable effects preclude their possible clinical application as "preconditioning-mimetic" agents (see Chapter 10). A related issue is specificity: Do these agonists and antagonists truly act exclusively at one locus of a specific messenger pathway without altering any other cellular function? Thus, rather than rely entirely upon data derived from the use of agonists and antagonists, our laboratory has approached the phenomenon of preconditioning from a different perspective: We have made use of empirical observations of infarct morphology to derive a mathematical explanation for the reduction in infarct size with preconditioning.

Mathematical evidence for protection via the nonischemic myocardium? (Figure 3)

Retrospective analysis of infarct size data from control and preconditioned rats subjected to 90 minutes of sustained coronary occlusion [41,46] revealed an interesting difference. In control animals, both infarct size (expressed as a percentage of the myocardium at risk of infarction) and the distance between the lateral boundary of the myocardium at risk and the edge of the infarct were independent of the size of the area at risk. In contrast, in hearts preconditioned by three 3-minute episodes of brief ischemia, *infarct size was dependent upon the extent of the myocardium at risk:* Infarct size increased and the lateral boundary decreased with increasing risk region (Figure 3). We used these data to formulate best-fit mathematical relationships between the extent of necrosis (AN), area at risk (AR), and the size of the lateral boundary of salvaged myocardium (denoted as "s"), the details of which are presented in reference [47]. As a result, we found that in preconditioned rat hears the relationships

$$AN/AR \propto 1 - [1/AR^2] \quad \text{and} \quad s \propto 1/AR$$

were highly consistent ($p = 0.004$) with the experimental data. In other words, these equations indicate that in preconditioned rat myocardium (1) the larger the risk region, the larger the infarct; and (2) the larger the risk region, the smaller the lateral boundary of salvage [47].

These relationships suggested to us that a protective substance might be entering the ischemic myocardium via the boundary of the risk region. Consequently, the declining efficacy of protection with increasing risk region might reflect an increasingly unfavorable change in the ratio of surface area to volume of myocardium at risk, and the concomitant decrease in the volume of noninfarcted tissue. Thus, our first hypothesis was that a *protective substance may be produced or activated throughout the heart by ischemic preconditioning.* Moreover, the inverse relationship between the lateral salvaged border and the area at risk, combined with the tendency for all preconditioned infarcts to be in the center of the area at risk, led to our second hypothesis, that *the protective substance(s) may be, in part, transported by diffusion.* We therefore applied classical diffusion equations to a simple two-dimensional model of the heart, in which we assumed production of a protective substance in the nonischemic tissue in an amount proportional to its area. This independent derivation based on the principles of simple diffusion produced relationships in good agreement with those derived from the experimental data [47].

Testing the model

Do these calculations simply represent an interesting exercise in mathematics, or does the mathematical model provide relevant insights into the possible mechanisms of preconditioning? We prospectively tested the derived concept that nonischemic tissue may play a role in ischemic preconditioning by performing brief transient ischemia in one region of the heart and then subjecting a different region of the heart to the sustained ischemic period. Specifically, anesthetized open-chest dogs underwent four repeated 5-minute occlusions of a branch of the circumflex (Cx) coronary artery, followed by 1 hour of sustained occlusion of the left anterior descending (LAD) coronary artery [48]. Infarct size in the LAD bed was significantly smaller in dogs subjected to brief Cx occlusion than in control animals subjected to 1 hour of LAD occlusion alone. In fact, the degree of infarct size reduction in this experiment was similar to that seen in conventional protocols involving either Cx preconditioning followed by Cx occlusion or LAD preconditioning followed by LAD occlusion [48]. As the reduction in infarct size could not be attributed to differences in hemodynamics or collateral perfusion between the groups, the data support the concept that ischemic preconditioning might be mediated, at least in part, by activating or producing factor(s) outside of the area subjected to brief ischemia/reperfusion.

The obvious question is, how does the nonischemic tissue "sense" ischemia in a remote region? Regional ischemia is associated with increases in interstitial adenosine concentration [49] and alterations in fatty acid metabolism [50] in remote nonischemic tissue, and in all likelihood results in global release of norepinephrine from cardiac nerve terminals. In addition, regional ischemia results in global left ventricular dilitation; in fact, in our "remote preconditioning" protocol, end-diastolic segment length in the LAD bed (assessed by sonomicrometry) increased modestly but significantly during the brief Cx occlusions [48]. As cellular stretch is known to play an important role in cellular communication and the regulation of transmembrane channels, this raised the possibility that stretch-activated mechanisms may play a role in ischemic preconditioning.

This concept was tested in a subsequent protocol by Ovize et al. [51], in which anesthetized dogs received either a rapid infusion of isotonic saline (500 ml at 38°C into the left atrium) or no intervention prior to a 1-hour period of sustained coronary occlusion. Rapid saline infusion resulted in a transient 15% increase in maximum segment length. This acute myocardial stretch in the absence of brief ischemia appeared to be cardioprotective: Infarct size in the volume-loaded dogs averaged 15% of the myocardium at risk, significantly smaller than the value of 32% of the risk region obtained in the control group. Ovize et al. further demonstrated that this protective effect of myocardial stretch could be blunted by the administration of gadolinium, an agent that is known to block stretch-activated ion channels in isolated cells and membranes. Moreover, gadolinium was also partially (but not completely) successful in attenuating the reduction in infarct size afforded by conventional ischemic preconditioning [51].

These studies of remote preconditioning and myocardial stretch do not explicitly validate the proposed mathematical model and do not identify the substance(s) responsible for the cardioprotective effects of brief ischemia. In fact, as discussed previously, we do not know whether the protective effects of conventional preconditioning, remote preconditioning, and/or stretch are regulated by a common mechanism(s). These protocols do, however, illustrate the potential use of this mathematical approach in the design of new experiments and the opening of new lines of investigation.

SUMMARY

To answer the question posed at the onset of this chapter: We have learned, first and foremost, that the observation of paradoxical cardioprotection by brief ischemia made by Murry, Jennings, and Reimer in 1986 [1] was not a spurious quirk. Rather, the unanimous observation of reduction in infarct size in preconditioned animals vs. controls has lead to the fundamental realization that the heart has the endogenous capacity to adapt to ischemia. Importantly, however, we have also learned that preconditioning is not a panacea: Its protective effects on myocyte viability are transient, it by no means attenuates all the deleterious consequences of ischemia/reperfusion, and it may even damage or decondition the myocardial collagen matrix. The reason *why* brief ischemia should delay myocyte death remains elusive, but may, at least in some species, involve activation of the adenosine A_1 receptor, opening of the K_{ATP} channel, and/or depletion of myocardial catecholamines. Moreover, evidence obtained from mathematical modeling suggests that the mediators(s) of ischemic preconditioning may be activated, produced, and/or transported throughout the heart by brief ischemia/reperfusion. Our current challenge is to build on the knowledge acquired since 1986 in an ongoing effort to elucidate the mechanism(s) responsible for ischemic preconditioning.

REFERENCES

1. Murry CE, Jennings RB, Reimer KA. 1986. Preconditioning with ischemia: A delay of lethal cell injury in ischemic myocardium. Circulation 74:1124–1136.
2. Ovize M, Przyklenk K, Kloner RA. 1992. Preconditioning does not attenuate myocardial stunning. Circulation 85:2247–2254.
3. Lawson CS, Coltart DJ, Hearse DJ. 1992. Ischemic preconditioning and reperfusion-induced arrhythmias: Reduction in vulnerability or delay in onset? Eur Heart J 13(Suppl):401 (abstr).
4. Defily DV, Chilian WM. 1993. Preconditioning protects coronary arteriolar endothelium from ischemia-reperfusion injury. Am J Physiol 265:H700–H706.
5. Bauer B, Simkhovich B, Kloner RA, Przyklenk K. 1993. Does preconditioning protect the coronary vasculature from subsequent ischemia/reperfusion injury? Circulation 88:659–672.
6. Zhao M, Zhang H, Robinson TF, Factor SM, Sonnenblick EH, Eng C. 1987. Profound structural alterations of the extracellular collagen matrix in postischemic dysfunctional ("stunned") but viable myocardium. J Am Coll Cardiol 10:1322–1334.
7. Whittaker P, Boughner DR, Kloner RA, Przyklenk K. 1991. Stunned myocardium and myocardial collagen damage: Differential effects of single and repeated occlusions. Am Heart J 121:434–441.

8. Whittaker P, Boughner DR, Kloner RA. 1991. Role of collagen in acute infarct expansion. Circulation 84:2123–2134.
9. Murry CE, Richard VJ, Reimer KA, Jennings RB. 1990. Ischemic preconditioning slows energy metabolism and delays ultrastructural damage during a sustained ischemic episode. Circ Res 66:913–931.
10. Hale SL, Kloner RA. 1992. Effect of ischemic preconditioning on regional myocardial flow in the rabbit heart. Coronary Artery Dis 3:133–140.
11. Knowlton AA, Brecher P, Apstein CS. 1991. Rapid expression of heat shock protein in the rabbit after brief cardiac ischemia. J Clin Invest 87:139–147.
12. Currie RW, Karmazyn M, Kloc M, Mailer K. 1988. Heat shock response is associated with enhanced postischemic ventricular recovery. Circ Res 63:543–549.
13. Yellon DM, Pasini E, Cargoni A, Marber MS, Latchman DS, Ferrari R. 1992. The protective role of heat stress in the ischemic and reperfusion rabbit myocardium. J Mol Cell Cardiol 24:895–907.
14. Marber MS, Latchman DS, Walker JM, Yellon DM. 1993. Cardiac stress protein elevation 24 hours following brief ischemia or heat stress is associated with resistance to myocardial infarction. Circulation, in press.
15. Currie RW, Tanguay RM, Kingma JG, Jr. 1993. Heat shock response and limitation of tissue necrosis during occlusion/reperfusion in rabbit hearts. Circulation 87:963–971.
16. Kloner RA, Przyklenk K, Whittaker P. 1989. Deleterious effects of oxygen radicals in ischemia/reperfusion: Resolved and unresolved issues. Circulation 80:1115–1127.
17. Iwamoto T, Miura T, Adachi T, Noto T, Ogawa T, Tsuchida A, Limura O. 1991. Myocardial infarct size-limiting effect of ischemic preconditioning was not attenuated by oxygen free-radical scavengers in the rabbit. Circulation 83:1015–1022.
18. Tanaka M, Fujiwara H, Yamasaki K. 1992. N-2-mercaptopropionyl glycine attenuates infarct size limiting effect of ischemic preconditioning. Circulation 86(Suppl I):I30 (abstr).
19. Omar BA, Hanson AK, Bose SK, McCord JM. 1991. Ischemic preconditioning is not mediated by free radicals in the isolated rabbit heart. Free Radical Biol Med 11:517–520.
20. Murry CE, Richard VJ, Jennings RB, Reimer KA. 1988. Preconditioning with ischemia: Is the effect mediated by free radical-induced myocardial stunning? Circulation 78(Suppl II):II77 (abstr).
21. Hoshida T, Kuzuya T, Fuji H, Yamashita N, Oe H, Hori M, Suzuki K, Tanaguchi N, Tada M. 1993. Sublethal ischemia alters myocardial antioxidant activity in canine heart. Am J Physiol 264:H33–H39.
22. Turrens JF, Thornton J, Barnard ML, Snyder S, Liu G, Downey JM. 1992. Protection from reperfusion injury by preconditioning hearts does not involve increased antioxidant defenses. Am J Physiol 262:H585–H589.
23. Liu GS, Thornton J, Van Winkle DM, Stanley AWH, Olsson RA, Downey JM. 1991. Protection against infarction afforded by preconditioning is mediated by A_1 adenosine receptors in rabbit heart. Circulation 84:350–356.
24. Thornton JD, Liu GS, Olsson RA, Downey JM. 1992. Intravenous pretreatment with A_1 selective adenosine analogues protects the heart against infarction. Circulation 85:659–665.
25. Alberts B, Bray D, Lewis J, Raff M, Roberts K, Watson JD (eds). Molecular Biology of the Cell, 2nd ed.; Garland Publishing, New York, 1989, pp. 693–708.
26. Green RD. 1991. Adenosine receptor, adenylate cyclase; relationships to pharmacological actions of adenosine. In Adenosine and Adenine Nucleotides as Regulators of Cellular Function, JW Phillis, ed. CRC Press, Boca Raton, FL, pp. 45–54.
27. Auchampach JA, Gross GJ. 1992. Activation of ATP-dependent potassium (K_{ATP}) channels by adenosine: A possible mechanism for ischemic preconditioning in dogs. Circulation 86(Suppl I):I340 (abstr).
28. Grover GJ, Sleph PG, Dzwonczyk S. 1992. Role of myocardial ATP-sensitive potassium channels in mediating preconditioning in the dog heart and their possible interaction with adenosine A_1 receptors. Circulation 86:1310–1316.
29. Schwarz ER, Mohri M, Sack S, Arras M. 1991. The role of adenosine and its A-1 receptor in ischemic preconditioning. Circulation 84:II191 (abstr).
30. Van Winkle DM, Chien GL, Wolff RA, Siofer BE, Davis RF. 1992. Intracoronary infusion of R-phenylisopropyl adenosine prior to ischemia/reperfusion reduces myocardial infarct size in swine. Circulation 86(Suppl I):I213 (abstr).

31. Li Y, Kloner RA. 1993. The cardioprotective effects of ischemic preconditioning are not mediated by adenosine receptors in rat hearts. Circulation 87:1642–1648.
32. Liu Y, Downey JM. 1992. Blocking adenosine receptors or ATP sensitive K^+ channels does not prevent preconditioning in rat heart. Circulation 86(Suppl I):I341 (abstr).
33. Gross GJ, Auchampach JA. 1992. Blockade of ATP-sensitive potassium channels prevents myocardial preconditioning in dogs. Circ Res 70:223–233.
34. Kirsch GE, Codina J, Birnbaumer L, Brown AM. 1990. Coupling of ATP-sensitive K^+ channels to A_1 receptors by G proteins in rat ventricular myocytes. Am J Physiol 259: H820–H826.
35. Rohmann S, Weygandt H, Schelling P, Lues I. 1992. ATP-sensitive potassium channel (K_{ATP}) opener bimakalim mimics preconditioning protection in swine. Circulation 86(Suppl I):I555.
36. Thornton JD, Thornton CS, Sterling DL, Downey JM. 1993. Blockade of ATP-sensitive potassium channels increases infarct size but does not prevent preconditioning in rabbit hearts. Circ Res 77:44–49.
37. Toombs CF, Moore TL, Shebuski RJ. 1993. Limitation of infarct size in the rabbit by ischaemic preconditioning is reversible with glibenclamide. Cardiovasc Res 27:617–622.
38. Grover GJ, Dzwonczyk S, Sleph PG. 1992. ATP-sensitive K^+ channel activation does not mediate preconditioning in isolated rat hearts. Circulation 86(Suppl I):I341 (abstr).
39. Locke-Winter CR, Winter CB, Nelson DW, Banerjee A. 1991. cAMP stimulation facilitates preconditioning against ischemia-reperfusion through norepinephrine and $alpha_1$ mechanisms. Circulation 84(Suppl II):II433 (abstr).
40. Vander Heide RS, Hill ML, Steenbergen C, Reimer KA, Jennings RB. 1991. Effect of reversible ischemia on mitochondrial ATPase activity in canine myocardium. Circulation 84(Suppl II):II192 (abstr).
41. Li Y, Whittaker P, Kloner RA. 1992. The transient nature of the effect of ischemic preconditioning on myocardial infarct size and ventricular arrhythmia. Am Heart J 123: 346–353.
42. Yellon DM, Alkhulaifi AM, Browne EE, Pugsley WB. 1992. Ischaemic preconditioning limits infarct size in the rat heart. Cardiovasc Res 26:983–987.
43. Shizukuda Y, Mallet RT, Lee SC, Downey HF. 1992. Hypoxic preconditioning of ischemic canine myocardium. Cardiovasc Res 26:534–542.
44. Ovize M, Przyklenk K, Kloner RA. 1992. Partial coronary stenosis is sufficient and complete reperfusion is mandatory for preconditioning the canine heart. Circ Res 71:1165–1173.
45. Bolli R, Zhu WX, Thornby JI, O'Neill PG, Roberts R. 1988. Time course and determinants of recovery of function after reversible ischemia in conscious dogs. Am J Physiol 254: H102–H114.
46. Li Y, Kloner RA. 1992. Cardioprotective effects of ischaemic preconditioning are not mediated by prostanoids. Cardiovasc Res 26:220–225.
47. Whittaker P, Li Y, Przyklenk K. 1993. Reduction of infarct size in vivo with ischemic preconditioning: Mathematical evidence for protection via non-ischemic tissue. Basic Res Cardiol, in press.
48. Przyklenk K, Bauer B, Ovize MO, Kloner RA, Whittaker P. 1993. Regional ischemic preconditioning protects remote virgin myocardium from subsequent sustained coronary occlusion. Circulation 87:893–899.
49. Dorheim TA, Hoffman A, Van Wylen DGL, Mentzner RM. 1991. Enhanced interstitial fluid adenosine attenuates myocardial stunning. Surgery 110:136–145.
50. Simkhovich BZ, Hale SL, Kloner RA. 1992. Effect of ischemic preconditioning on carnitine-linked metabolism in the rabbit heart. Coronary Artery Dis 3:141–147.
51. Ovize M, Przyklenk K, Kloner RA. 1992. Myocardial dilatation, in the absence of ischemia, preconditions the canine heart. Circulation 86(Suppl I):I32 (abstr).

III. ISCHEMIC PRECONDITIONING: LABORATORY CURIOSITY OR CLINICAL PROMISE?

10. IS PRECONDITIONING RELEVANT TO CLINICAL MEDICINE?

ROBERT A. KLONER and KARIN PRZYKLENK

INTRODUCTION

Previous chapters in this book have detailed the phenomenon of ischemic preconditioning in a host of animal models. The obvious question is, does preconditioning have any relevance for the clinical cardiologist? The purpose of the present chapter is to review the evidence that preconditioning and adaptation to myocardial ischemia might occur in humans and to review potential clinical applications of preconditioning as therapy for ischemic syndromes.

EVIDENCE OF PRECONDITIONING IN HUMANS

Preconditioning during angioplasty procedures?

One of the first studies to demonstrate that ischemic preconditioning might occur in humans was that of Deutsch and coworkers [1]. These investigators studied the response of the human heart to repetitive brief episodes of ischemia induced by angioplasty. Twelve patients underwent two sequential 90-second angioplasty balloon inflations of the left anterior descending coronary artery. The second balloon inflation was associated with less anginal intensity (Table 1), less ST-segment deviation on the electrocardiogram (0.44 mV vs. 0.21 mV), less production of myocardial lactate (Figure 1), and lower mean pulmonary artery pressures when compared with the first balloon inflation. In addition, although cardiac vein flow rapidly fell and

Table 1. Clinical, hemodynamic, and electrocardiographic responses to percutaneous transluminal coronary angioplasty

Patient	CP1	CP2	ST1 (mV)	ST2 (mV)	MAP1 (mmHg)	MAP2 (mmHg)	HR1 (beats/min)	HR2 (beats/min)
1	10	5	1.0	0.5	88	90	64	60
2	9	6	0.7	0.2	100	96	68	70
3	8	3	0.7	0.3	92	90	76	70
4	10	4	0.6	0.4	94	94	60	60
5	7	2	0.8	0.5	84	88	58	56
6	8	3	0.6	0.3	90	90	66	68
7	9	3	0.5	0.3	102	95	78	84
Mean	8.7	3.8[a]	0.7	0.35[b]	93	92[c]	67	67[c]
SEM	±1.0	±0.8	±0.2	±0.1	±4.2	±2.3	±2.6	±2.5

CP, anginal score (based on 0–10 visual analogue scale); 1, inflation 1; 2, inflation 2; ST, ST-segment shift; MAP, mean systemic arterial pressure; HR, heart rate.
[a] $p = 0.001$ vs. inflation 1.
[b] $p = 0.005$ vs. inflation 1.
[c] p = NS vs. inflation 1.
Reprinted from Deutsch et al. [1], with permission from the American Heart Association.

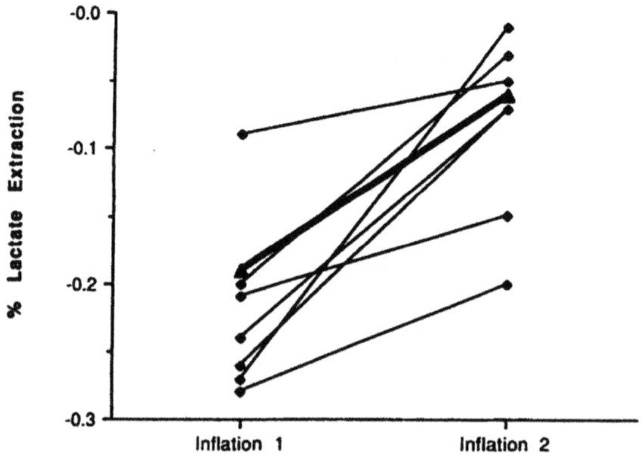

Figure 1. Transmyocardial lactate extraction during percutaneous transluminal coronary angioplasty in seven patients. Fractional lactate extraction during the first inflation (−11 ± 3%) was significantly lower than that during the second inflation (−3 ± 2%). Triangles and thick line indicate mean values. Reprinted from Deutsch et al. [1] with permission of the American Heart Association.

remained reduced throughout both sequential balloon inflations, cardiac vein flow was lower during the second inflation than during the first, despite the fact that the rate-pressure product was similar during both of the brief ischemic episodes. The authors concluded that the lessened ischemic response during the second balloon inflation was evidence that the myocardium had been preconditioned by the first inflation. The fact that cardiac vein flow was lower during the second inflation than the first suggested that this apparent adaptation to ischemia was not due to an increase in collateral flow.

Two recent reports have confirmed this concept of preconditioning during angioplasty [2,3] and have further explored the question of whether recruitment of collateral blood flow might play a role in adaptation to acute ischemia [2]. For example, Cribier and colleagues [2] studied 17 patients in whom five balloon inflations, each 60–180 seconds in duration, were performed. In addition to measuring chest pain, intracoronary ST-segment elevation, hemodynamics, ejection fraction, and length of the hypokinetic zone by angiography, the extent of collateral filling was also graded. Similar to the study by Deutsch and coworkers [4], Cribier and colleagues reported that the severity of chest pain and the degree of ST-segment elevation was decreased with sequential balloon inflations (Figures 2–4). In addition, the elevation in left ventricular end diastolic pressure (LVEDP) was less pronounced during the fifth inflation than during the second, and the deterioration in ejection fraction was attenuated during the fifth inflation when compared with the second. The degree of collateral filling, determined by a semiquantitative scoring system, increased in 10 patients between the first and second inflations, but remained unchanged in the remaining seven patients. Mean coronary artery occlusion pressure, an index of the extent of collateral perfusion, was significantly higher during the fourth (36 mmHg) compared with the first (31 mmHg) balloon inflation.

Thus, the study by Cribier et al. [2] confirmed the concept that human myocardium might be preconditioned by brief episodes of transient ischemia. However, in contrast to results obtained in the experimental setting [4] — and in contrast to the data of Deutsch et al. [1] — Cribier and colleagues

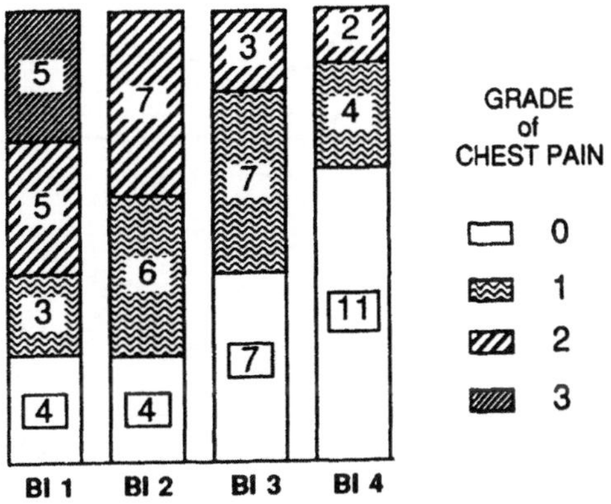

Figure 2. Decrease in chest pain with four sequential balloon inflations. Chest pain was graded from 0–3 at 120 seconds after the onset of each balloon inflation (BI), according to the intensity of discomfort. The number of patients with each grade appears in the squares. Reprinted with permission from Cribier et al. [2].

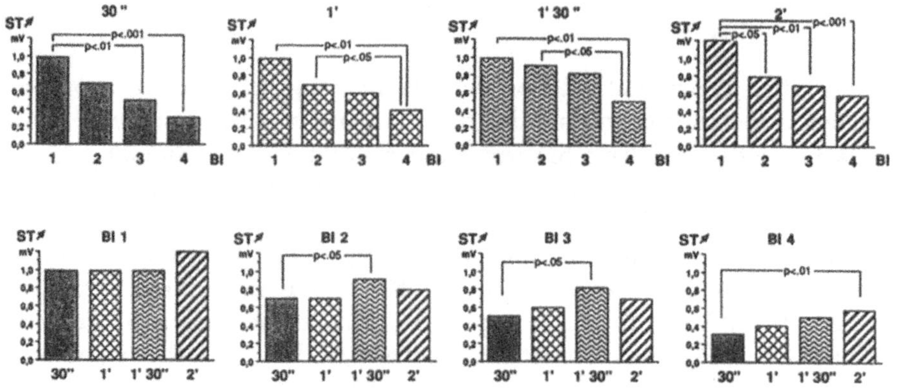

Figure 3. Pattern of evolution of intracoronary ST-segment elevation (ST↗) as recorded every 30 seconds up to 120 seconds during four sequential balloon inflations. **Upper panel**: Comparison of ST shift at a similar time during each of the four balloon inflations (BI), showing a progressive decrease in ST-segment elevation. **Lower panel**: ST shift in relation to time, indicating a decreased rate of ST-segment elevation with successive coronary occlusion. All statistically significant differences are indicated. Reprinted with permission from Cribier et al. [2].

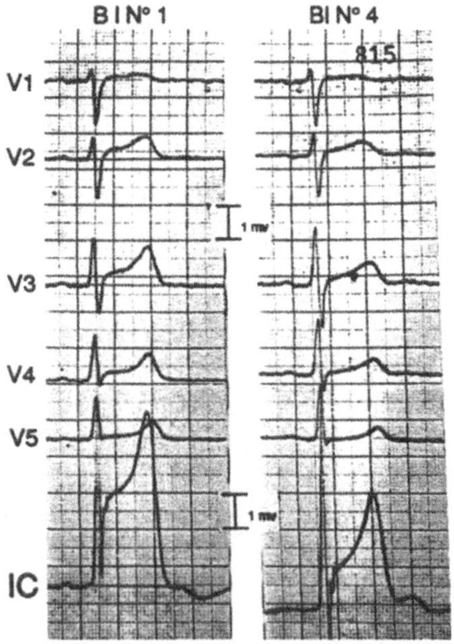

Figure 4. Representative example of ST-segment changes observed in one patient at 120 seconds after the onset of the first and fourth balloon inflations (BI) in surface electrocardiographic (ECG) leads V_1 to V_5 and in the intracoronary (IC) ECG. In the surface ECG, the maximal ST elevation was noted in precordial lead V_3; it was measured to be 0.4 mV at the first and 0.2 mV at the fourth coronary occlusion. In comparison, in the intracoronary ECG, a dramatic ST elevation of 2.3 mV was observed during the first balloon inflation, but ST elevation was only 0.9 mV during the fourth balloon inflation. Reprinted with permission from Cribier et al. [2].

observed acute recruitment of collateral channels with sequential episodes of myocardial ischemia. The relationship between adaptation to ischemia and recruitment of collateral vessels is, however, unclear, as some patients demonstrated decreased evidence of ischemia with repetitive balloon inflations, even in the *absence* of improved collateral blood flow [2].

Not all angioplasty studies, however, have supported the concept that preconditioning occurs in humans. One consideration is that the duration of balloon inflation may be an important determinant of this phenomenon: In studies of very brief sequential balloon inflations of less than 1 minute, preconditioning apparently does not occur [5–7]. For example, in one report patients underwent two control balloon inflations of 60 seconds or less, and the presence of angina and ST-segment shifts was similar during both inflations [6].

A preliminary report by Denys et al. [8] suggested that some, but not all, patients showed an increase in time to maximal ST elevation between a first and second balloon inflation. However, they concluded that this difference was due to ischemia after balloon insertion but prior to the first angioplasty. In other words, the deflated angioplasty balloon crossing a narrow obstruction prior to the first inflation was enough to further decrease blood flow, causing a longer total duration of ischemia than that associated with the second inflation of the then-dilated lesion. A study by DeBruyne et al. [9] showed less angina after a fourth 60-second angioplasty inflation when compared with the first balloon inflation. This was not, however, associated with differences in left ventricular function. The authors concluded that the lack of effect of repetitive occlusion on left ventricular function suggested that angioplasty was not a good model of myocardial preconditioning. However, despite apparent benefits of preconditioning on recovery of function in isolated heart preparations, our own results in the experimental laboratory have failed to observe any beneficial effect of preconditioning on segmental wall motion in an in vivo regional ischemia model [10; see also Chapter 3].

Thus, most angioplasty studies have suggested that with repetitive balloon inflations there is progressively less angina and fewer ECG changes during ischemia. In the authors' opinion, this probably does reflect "true" preconditioning as defined in the experimental laboratory, although the exact mechanism(s) for this apparent adaptation remain to be established.

Does preinfarction angina protect the myocardium?

There is no question that patients may experience brief episodes of ischemia prior to acute myocardial infarction [11]. Is it possible that these brief ischemic events might precondition the myocardium, and thereby lessen ischemic damage? The answer to this question is not yet known. However, Ovize et al. [10] provided experimental evidence that repeated formation and dislodgement of platelet thrombi (mimicking unstable angina) can precondition the canine heart. Specifically, anesthetized dogs were subjected to partial

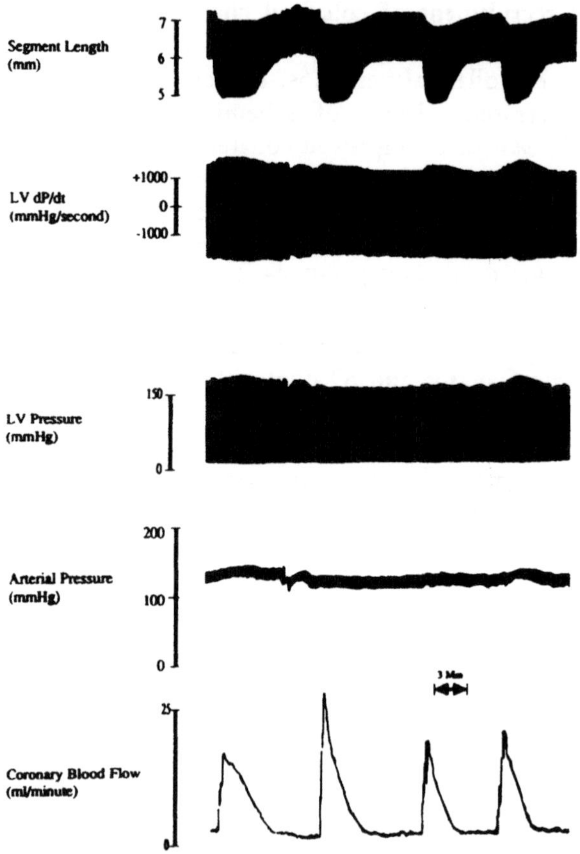

Figure 5. Representative recording from dog with cyclic flow variations. Note progressive decline in coronary blood flow followed by abrupt restoration of flow after thrombus dislodgement and embolization. These episodes did not significantly influence arterial pressure. In contrast, thrombus formation clearly induced increases in end-diastolic and end-systolic lengths that returned to previous values after restoration of coronary blood flow. The first derivative of left ventricular pressure (LV dP/dt), an index of global left ventricular (LV) function, paralleled alterations in segment shortening. Reprinted from Ovize et al. [10] with permission from the American Heart Association.

coronary artery stenosis at a site of endothelial injury, resulting in platelet activation, adherence, and dislodgement, and thereby producing cyclic variations in coronary blood flow (Figure 5). A 30-minute period of cyclic flow variation (or CFV) "protected" the myocardium from a subsequent 1-hour episode of sustained coronary occlusion: Infarct size was significantly smaller in the CFV group than in control animals that received no intervention prior to sustained ischemia (Figure 6). Thus, the scenario of endothelial injury, coronary stenosis, and cyclical thrombus formation, all components of un-

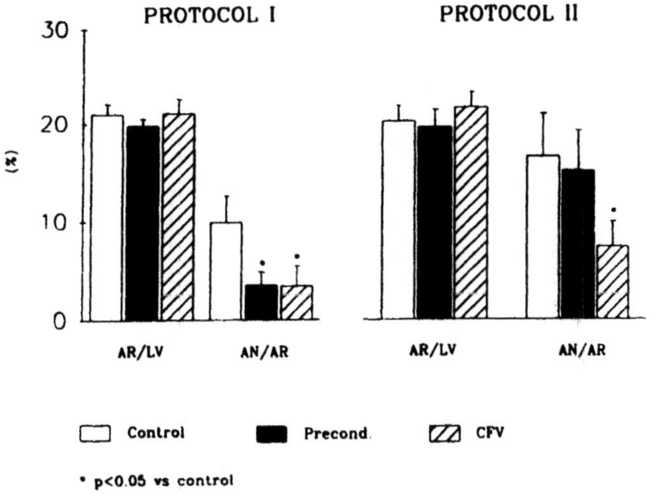

Figure 6. Effect of cyclic flow variations (CFV) on myocardial infarct size. Bar graphs of effects of CFV, mechanical preconditioning (Precond.), and no intervention (control) on infarct size after 60 (protocol 1) and 90 minutes (protocol 2) of sustained coronary occlusion. Protocol 1: The area at risk (AR), expressed as percentage of the left ventricle (LV), was similar in all groups. Area of necrosis (AN), expressed as percentage of AR, was significantly reduced in both CFV and preconditioned groups ($p < 0.05$ vs. control). Protocol 2: The AR was same in all groups. Only CFV dogs experienced significant reduction in infarct size ($p < 0.05$ vs. control). Reprinted from Ovize et al. [10] with permission of the American Heart Association.

stable angina, preconditioned or protected the heart from subsequent prolonged ischemia in this canine model.

The effect of preinfarction angina on outcome following myocardial infarction had been the subject of several recent clinical reports. In one study, Hirai et al. [12] found that patients who experienced angina for more than 1 week before the onset of permanent coronary occlusion had a higher left ventricular ejection fraction (measured an average of 37 days after infarction) and superior wall motion in the infarct-related zone than both patients without preinfarction angina and patients in whom preinfarction angina occurred only within 1 week prior to infarction. Specifically, regional segment shortening averaged 10 ± 3%, −1 ± 2%, and 1 ± 2% in the three groups, respectively (Figures 7 and 8). Coronary collateral channels (visualized by angiography) were present during the acute phase of myocardial infarction in 67%, 20%, and 25% of patients who had preinfarction angina for greater than 1 week, those who had angina within 1 week of infarction, and those without preinfarction angina, respectively. Moreover, semiquantitative scoring of collateral perfusion revealed that the collateral index was higher in patients with preinfarction angina for greater than 1 week (score of 1.4) when compared with the other two groups (scores of 0.4 and 0.5, respectively; Figure 9).

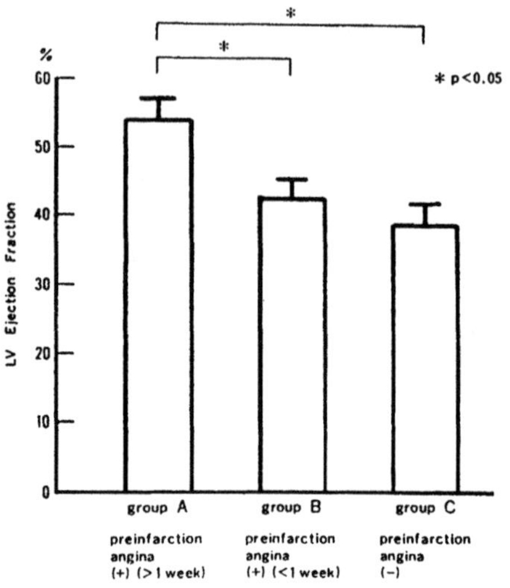

Figure 7. Bar graph of left ventricular ejection fraction in patients with angina for >1 week before infarction: patients with angina within 1 week before infarction and patients without preinfarction angina. Error bars denote standard error of the mean in each group. Reprinted with permission from Hirai et al. [12].

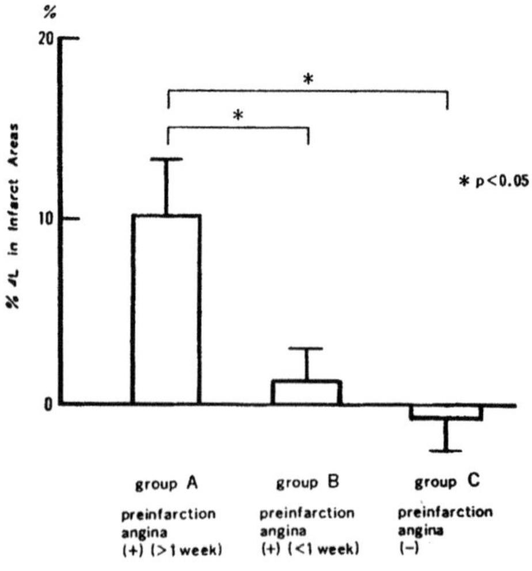

Figure 8. Bar graph of regional segment shortening in the infarct area in the three groups described in Figure 7. Reprinted with permission from Hirai et al. [12].

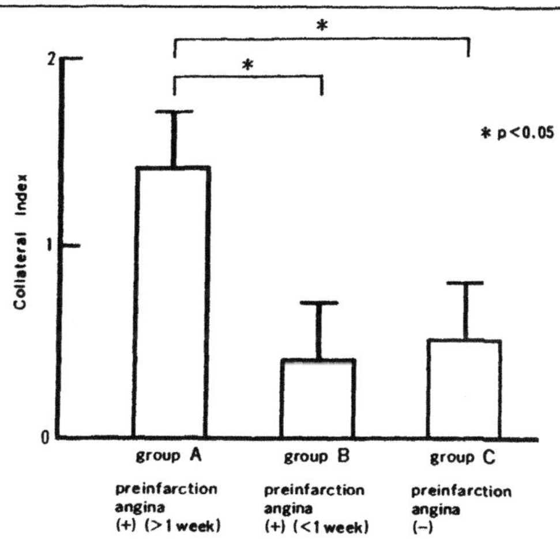

Figure 9. Bar graph of collateral index in the three groups described in Figure 7 at the time of acute myocardial infarction. Reprinted with permission from Hirai et al. [12].

Thus, angina for more than 1 week prior to infarction was associated with both improved collateral perfusion and improved ventricular function, leading the authors to conclude the "repetitive myocardial ischemic stimuli exerted a beneficial effect on the preservation of myocardial function." However, two lines of evidence suggest that the improved wall motion in this group probably does not represent "true" preconditioning (i.e., the reduction in infarct size as defined in experimental protocols). Specifically, data obtained from the in vivo canine model indicates that (1) preconditioning is not associated with (or caused by) an improvement in collateral blood flow [4]; and, in fact, (2) preconditioning is not accompanied by an acute improvement in regional wall motion [10]. Whether patients who experienced angina only within 1 week of infarction developed smaller infarcts, but exhibited similar dysfunction when compared to patients without preinfarction angina, is unknown. This study does, however, make the important observation that repetitive episodes of ischemia occurring over an extended period of time can lead to an adaptive process — in this case, the development of collateral vessels — which then appear to serve as a protective mechanism during infarction.

Muller et al. [13] also observed a less complicated short-term clinical course in patients who had a history of angina for more than 1 week prior to infarction when compared with patients without angina (Table 2). Patients with antecedent chest pain had a significantly lower rate of reocclusion of the infarct-related artery after reperfusion therapy (8.2% vs. 13.6% in patients without antecedent chest pain) and demonstrated a nonsignificant trend towards lower in-hospital mortality [4.6% vs. 7.2%]. Although the reasons for

Table 2. Clinical and angiographic outcome

Outcome	No prior angina	Prior angina
Nadir serum fibrinogen (gm/l)	1.0 (1.7, 6.9)	0.9 (1.5, 5.2)
Peak FDPs (μg/ml)[a]	210 (770, 2700)	210 (900, 2700)
Reocclusion (%)[b]	13.6	8.2
Recurrent ischemia (%)	24.5	17.1
IRA at discharge (%)		
Patent (<50%)	49.7	49.5
Patent (51%–99%)	9.0	8.7
Occluded	7.7	6.1
Bypass graft	19.6	20.9
Patient died	7.2	4.6
Unknown	6.8	10.2
Pulmonary edema (%)	12.6	11.7
CABG (%)		
Emergency	4.9	6.1
Urgent	6.0	4.6
Elective	10.3	11.2
Death (in hospital, %)[c]	7.2	4.6
Two-year survival after discharge (%)	98.5	94.2
Cumulative 2-year survival (%)	90.2	89.1

CABG, coronary artery bypass graft surgery; FDPs, fibrinogen degradation products; IRA, infarct-related artery.
[a] Median (25th, 75th percentiles)
[b] $p = 0.048$.
[c] $p = 0.21$.
Reprinted with permission from Muller et al. [13].

the better short-term course in patients with prior angina is unknown, the authors speculated that enhanced collateral perfusion, preconditioning, prior therapy with beta or calcium blockers, or intrinsic differences in the thrombolytic systems between the groups of patients may all have played a role.

Ottani et al. [14] compared patients suffering a first anterior myocardial infarction treated with thrombolytic agents who either did or did not develop prodromal angina within 24 hours of the onset of symptoms. Infarct size, determined by release of creatine kinase and the number of hypokinetic segments detected by left ventricular angiography, was significantly smaller in the group with prodromal angina, leading the investigators to conclude that prodromal angina had "preconditioned" these infarcts.

In contrast to the studies by Hirai et al. [12], Muller et al. [13] and Ottani et al. [14], Behar and colleagues [15] concluded that angina pectoris preceding a first acute myocardial infarction may be associated with a poor prognosis. Of the 4166 patients enrolled in this study, 43% had angina pectoris for more than 1 month prior to infarction. Both in-hospital as well as 5-year postdischarge mortality rates were significantly higher among patients with chronic angina when compared to patients without previous angina (Figure 10). Multiple logistic function analysis revealed that angina pectoris was a predictor of increased hospital mortality, independent of age, site of infarction,

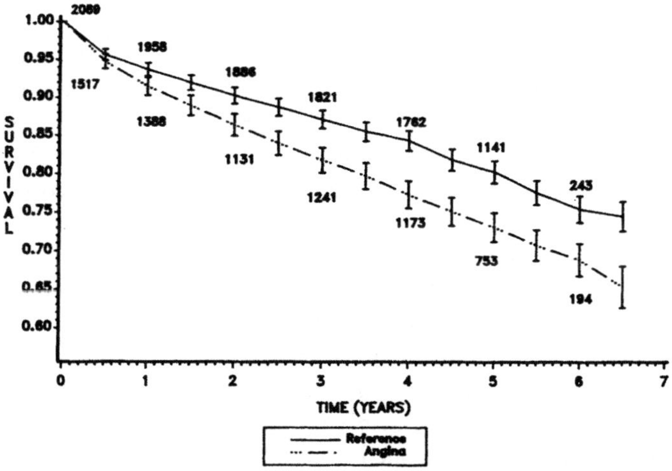

Figure 10. Actuarial survival curves of hospital survivors with and without antecedent angina preceding first acute myocardial infarction. Reprinted with permission from Behar et al. [15].

diabetes, and heart failure. A potential explanation for this result is that patients with chronic angina may have had more extensive coronary artery disease. Another negative study was recently reported by Karagounis et al. [16]. In this case regional wall motion abnormalities and ejection fractions were similar in patients with and without a history of angina prior to myocardial infarction. Ruocco et al. [17] observed that in the Thrombolysis in Myocardial Infarction Phase II (TIMI II) trial, antecedent angina identified patients at increased risk for recurrent in-hospital chest pain and recurrent infarction at 1 year. Patients with a history of angina before their infarction also had more severe residual atherosclerotic narrowing following thrombolysis and a greater frequency of multivessel coronary artery disease. A recent report from the Framingham study [18] showed that 21% of men and 25% of women had preexisting angina pectoris at any time prior to myocardial infarction. Patients were followed for 34 years after their initial infarction. Preexisting angina increased the risk of death due to coronary heart disease and a second myocardial infarction by 50% in men. Preexisting angina increased the risk of a second myocardial infarction by 70% in women. Thus, there is clearly no consensus concerning the question of whether preinfarction angina is "protective" or deleterious. To date, definitive clinical evidence that preinfarction angina acutely protects or preconditions the heart is lacking. However, most studies have not specifically determined the effect of angina immediately prior to infarction (that is, within 24–48 hours), which would more closely approximate preconditioning ischemia described in experimental models.

Can preconditioning reduce ischemic damage in patients with severe stable angina?

It is conceivable that preconditioning might play a role in reducing the amount of ischemic damage that occurs in patients with frequent episodes of severe angina and/or silent ischemia. While this issue has not been studied directly, there is some indirect evidence supporting this concept. Nørregaard-Hansen et al. [19] assessed serum levels of myoglobin and creatine kinase in patients with severe stable angina. All patients had positive exercise tolerance tests and angiographic evidence of significant coronary artery disease. Ambulatory electrocardiographic ST-segment monitoring revealed 47 episodes of ischemia (the majority of which were silent) in a subgroup of patients, with the total duration of ischemia ranging from to 599 to 804 minutes. Despite these multiple ischemic episodes, there was no release of myoglobin, CK, or CK-MB. These data raise the possibility that multiple episodes of ischemia "preconditioned" these hearts and prevented cumulative damage, but additional investigations are needed to confirm this observation.

POTENTIAL THERAPEUTIC APPLICATIONS OF PRECONDITIONING IN THE CLINICAL SETTING

Despite the ongoing controversy concerning the existence of ischemic preconditioning in patients with coronary artery disease, the beneficial results obtained in the experimental setting have lead investigators to speculate on potential therapeutic applications of this phenomenon. For example, it is conceivable that hearts that are subjected to a planned absence of flow, such as donor hearts removed for transplantation or hearts placed on cardiopulmonary bypass, might undergo prophylactic ischemic preconditioning prior to sustained ischemia. Theoretically, preconditioning could be induced in these hearts by intermittent aortic cross-clamping or brief (1–2-minute) transient occlusion of the coronary arteries. Of note, intermittent aortic clamping, rather than standard cardioplegia, is a method currently used by some cardiothoracic surgeons. Alternatively, if the mechanism for preconditioning is elucidated, "preconditioning-mimetic" agents might be administered prophylactically prior to transplantation or bypass. In this regard, some [20], but not all [21], studies have suggested that adenosine or adenosine agonists might serve as preconditioning-mimetic agents (see Chapter 8). Secondly, pharmacologic agents that mimic or simulate ischemic preconditioning might also be used for unplanned ischemic events, such as angina pectoris or myocardial infarction; that is, it is possible that an agent that simulates preconditioning might be administered prophylactically to patients with coronary artery disease who are at risk of suffering major cardiac events. While agents such as adenosine had been considered to be a potential preconditioning-mimetic agents [20], one preliminary study in which dipyridamole (an agent that increases adenosine levels) was administered as adjunctive therapy to thrombolysis failed to demonstrate any further beneficial effect on left ventricular function or infarct size [22]. Finally, several studies using the rat model [23–25] (and some reports in the canine model [26]) have found that brief episodes of preconditioning ischemia can reduce the incidence of ventricular arrhythmias during subsequent sustained coronary artery occlusion and reperfusion. If the mechanism(s) responsible for the antiarrhythmic effects of preconditioning can be determined, then it is conceivable that preconditioning or preconditioning-mimetic drugs might also be used as antiarrhythmic therapy. It must be stressed, however, that the potential therapeutic role of preconditioning is, at present, purely speculative.

OTHER ADAPTIVE PROCESSES

While this chapter has focused on preconditioning as an adaptive process of the heart to ischemia, it is important to remember that other adaptive processes also exist. For example, myocardial hibernation is thought to represent an adaptive process whereby the heart downregulates its metabolism in the setting of chronic low blood flow in order to maintain myocyte viability [27,28]. Patients with hibernating myocardium exhibit severe coronary artery stenosis, resulting in chronic left ventricular wall motion abnormalities, which may persist for months or years. The myocytes distal to the stenosis are not, however, necrotic, as demonstrated by the normal or enhanced glucose uptake and metabolism of this tissue detected by positron emission tomography [29]. Moreover, revascularization of hibernating myocardium by either coronary artery bypass surgery or angioplasty results in an eventual improvement in contractile performance. A second form of adaptation is the development of coronary collateral vessels in the setting of ongoing ischemia. Some investigators believe that collateral vessels may preserve myocyte viability during subsequent coronary artery occlusion [12]. However, the collateral vessels do not usually prevent ischemia per se, and patients with extensive collateralization between coronary artery beds also usually have extensive coronary artery disease.

It is important to note that both the phenomenon of the hibernating myocardium and development of new collateral vessels differ from preconditioning in that the first two are consequences of chronic (days to months) low blood flow, whereas preconditioning is an acute consequences of brief transient ischemia. Nevertheless, all three phenomena appear to be protective.

SUMMARY

There is no doubt that brief episodes of transient ischemia protect the rat, rabbit, dog, and swine heart from subsequent sustained coronary occlusion. The obvious question is, can we extrapolate these observations to the clinical realm? There is some evidence (albeit equivocal) for adaptation to ischemia both during angioplasty procedures and in patients with preinfarction angina. In addition, a very recent study [30] suggested that intermittent cross-clamping slowed ATP depletion in patients undergoing coronary artery bypass surgery, implying that it may be possible to precondition the human heart. Whether these examples of adaptation truly represent preconditioning as defined in the experimental laboratory remains to be elucidated. Nonetheless, these data have fostered hope and speculation that the phenomenon of preconditioning may be exploited and used to develop therapies for a wide range of cardiovascular disorders.

REFERENCES

1. Deutsch E, Berger M, Kussmaul WG, Hirshfeld JW, Herrmann HC, Laskey WL. 1990. Adaptation to ischemia during percutaneous transluminal coronary angioplasty. Clinical, hemodynamic, and metabolic features. Circulation 82:2044–2051.
2. Cribier A, Korsatz L, Koning R, Rath P, Gamra H, Stix G, Merchant S, Chan C, Letac B. 1992. Improved myocardial ischemic response and enhanced collateral circulation with long repetitive coronary occlusion during angioplasty: A prospective study. J Am Coll Cardiol 20:578–586.
3. Heibig J, Bolli R, Harris S. 1989. Initial coronary occlusion improves tolerance to subsequent prolonged balloon inflations. Cathet Cardiovasc Diagn 16:99–102.
4. Murry CE, Jennings RB, Reimer KA. 1986. Preconditioning with ischemia: A delay of lethal cell injury in ischemic myocardium. Circulation 75:1124–1136.
5. Hill JA, Feldman RL, MacDonald RG, Pepine CJ. 1985. Coronary artery collateral visualization during acute coronary occlusion. Am J Cardiol 55:1216–1218.
6. Feldman RL, MacDonald RG, Hill JA, et al. 1986. Effect of propranolol on myocardial ischemia during acute coronary occlusion. Circulation 73:727–733.
7. Zalewski A, Goldberg S, Cervan JD, Slysh S, Maroko PR. 1986. Myocardial protection during transient coronary artery occlusion in man: Beneficial effects of regional beta adrenergic blockade. Circulation 73:734–739.
8. Denys BG, Lee J, Reddy PS, Uretsky BF. 1992. Is there adaptation to ischemia during PTCA? Eur Heart J 13:246.
9. DeBruyne B, Vantrimpont PJ, Goetua SM, Stockbrockx J, Paulus WJ. 1992. Can coronary angioplasty serve as a model of myocardial preconditioning? Circulation 86(Suppl I):I378.
10. Ovize M, Kloner RA, Hale SL, Przyklenk K. 1992. Coronary cyclic flow variations "precondition" ischemic myocardium. Circulation 85:779–789.
11. Deanfield JE, Selwyn AP, Chierchia S, Maseri A, Ribeiro P, Krikler S, Morgan M. 1983. Myocardial ischemia during daily life in patients with stable angina: Its relation to symptoms and heart rate changes. Lancet 1:753–758.
12. Hirai T, Fujita M, Yamanishi K, Ohno A, Miwa K, Sasayama S. 1992. Significance of preinfarction angina for preservation of left ventricular function in acute myocardial infarction. Am Heart J 124:19–23.
13. Muller DWM, Topol EJ, Califf RM, Sigmon KN, Gorman L, George BS, Kereiakes DJ, Lee KL, Ellis SG, and TAMI Study Group. 1990. Relationship between antecedent angina pectoris and short term prognosis after thrombolytic therapy for acute myocardial infarction. Am Heart J 119:224–231.
14. Ottani F, Galvani M, Ferrini D, Morgagni GL, Pettini A, Sorbello F, Rusticali F. 1993. Ischemic preconditioning: Prodromal angina limits myocardial infarct size. J Am Coll Cardiol 21:149A.
15. Behar S, Reicher RH, Abinader E, et al. 1992. The prognostic significance of angina pectoris preceding the occurrence of a first acute myocardial infarction in 4166 consecutive hospitalized patients. Am Heart J 123:1481–1486.
16. Karagounis LA, Anderson JL, Becker LC, and TEAM 5 Investigators. 1993. Does chronic ischemic preconditioning limit infarct size in patients treated with fibrinolytics for acute myocardial infarction? J Am Coll Cardiol 21:150A.
17. Ruocco NA, Bergelson BA, Jacobs AK, Frederick MM, Faxon DP, Ryan TJ. 1992. Invasive versus conservative strategy after thrombolytic therapy for acute myocardial infarction in patients with antecedent angina. A report from thrombolysis in myocardial infarction phase II (TIMI II). J Am Coll Cardiol 20:1445–1451.

18. Cupples LA, Gagnon DR, Wong ND, Ostfeld AM, Kannel WB. 1993. Preexisting cardiovascular conditions and long-term prognosis after initial myocardial infarction. The Framingham Study. Am Heart J 125:863–872.
19. Nørregaard-Hansen K, Egstrup K, Nielsen JR, Jørgensen PJ, Petersen PH, Haghfelt T, Hørder M. 1993. Lack of indication of myocardial cell damage after myocardial ischaemia in patients with severe stable angina. Eur Heart J 13:188–193.
20. Liu GS, Thornton J, VanWinkle DM, Stanley AWH, Olsson RA, Downey JM. 1991. Protection against infarction afforded by preconditioning is mediated by A_1-adenosine receptors in the rabbit heart. Circulation 84:350–356.
21. Hale SL, Bellows SD, Hammerman H, Kloner RA. 1992. High dose intracoronary adenosine does not mimic ischemic preconditioning in the rabbit. Submitted.
22. Van de Werf F, Janssens L, Brzostek T, De Geest H. 1992. Effects of increased myocardial adenosine concentrations in patients with acute myocardial infarction receiving thrombolytic therapy. Circulation 86(Suppl I):I803.
23. Shiki K, Hearse DJ. 1987. Preconditioning of ischemic myocardium: Reperfusion-induced arrhythmias. Am J Physiol 253:H1470–H1476.
24. Hagar JM, Hale SL, Kloner RA. 1991. Effect of preconditioning ischemia on reperfusion arrhythmias after coronary artery occlusion and reperfusion in the rat. Circ Res 68:61–68.
25. Li Y, Whittaker P, Kloner RA. 1992. The transient nature of the effect of ischemic preconditioning on myocardial infarct size and ventricular arrhythmias. Am Heart J 123: 346–353.
26. Vegh A, Szekeres L, Parratt JR. 1990. Protective effects of preconditioning of the ischemic myocardium involves cyclooxygenose products. Cardiovasc Res 24:1020–1023.
27. Kloner RA, Przyklenk K, Rahimtoola S. Braunwald E. 1990. Myocardial stunning and hibernation: Mechanisms and clinical implications. In Heart Disease: Update 11, E Braunwald, ed. W.B. Saunders, Philadelphia, pp. 241–256.
28. Fedele FA, Gerwitz H, Capone RJ, Sharaf B, Most AS. 1988. Metabolic response to prolonged reduction of myocardial blood flow distal to a severe coronary artery stenosis. Circulation 78:729–738.
29. Tillisch J, Brunken R, Marshall R, Schwaiger M, Mandelkerm M, Phelps M, Schelbert H. 1986. Reversibility of cardiac wall-motion abnormalities predicted by positron tomography. N Engl J Med 314:884–888.
30. Yellon DM, Alkhulaifi AM, Pugsley WB. 1993. Preconditioning the human myocardium. Lancet 342:276–277.

INDEX

GPSR Compliance

The European Union's (EU) General Product Safety Regulation (GPSR) is a set of rules that requires consumer products to be safe and our obligations to ensure this.

If you have any concerns about our products, you can contact us on ProductSafety@springernature.com

In case Publisher is established outside the EU, the EU authorized representative is:

Springer Nature Customer Service Center GmbH
Europaplatz 3
69115 Heidelberg, Germany

Batch number: 10755292

Printed by Printforce, the Netherlands